Recovery Recipes For

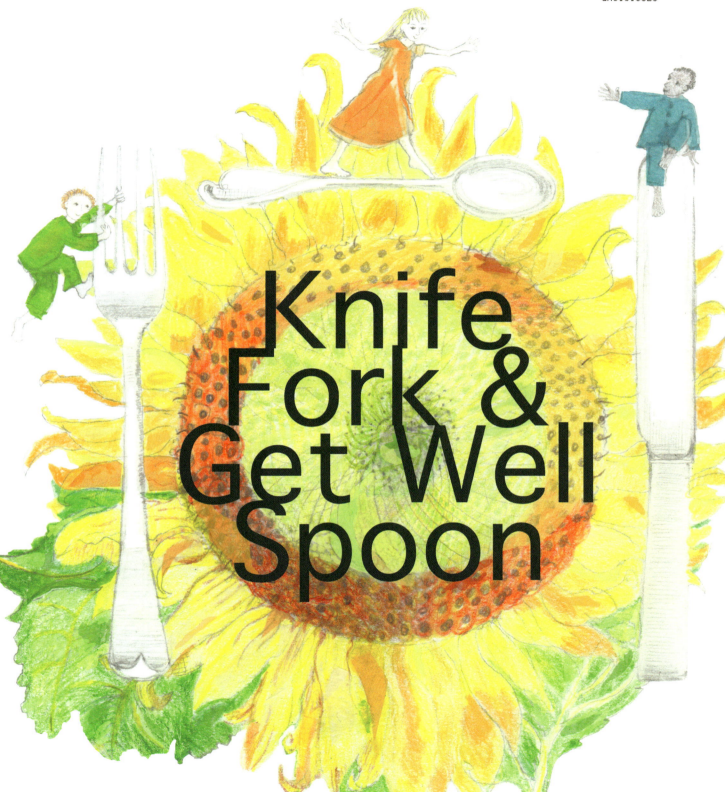

Knife Fork & Get Well Spoon

Victoria Kell & Aletta Ritchie

AuthorHouse™ UK Ltd.
1663 Liberty Drive
Bloomington, IN 47403 USA
www.authorhouse.co.uk
Phone: 0800.197.4150

Published by AuthorHouse 09/09/2014

ISBN: 978-1-4969-7925-4 (sc)
ISBN: 978-1-4969-7926-1 (e)

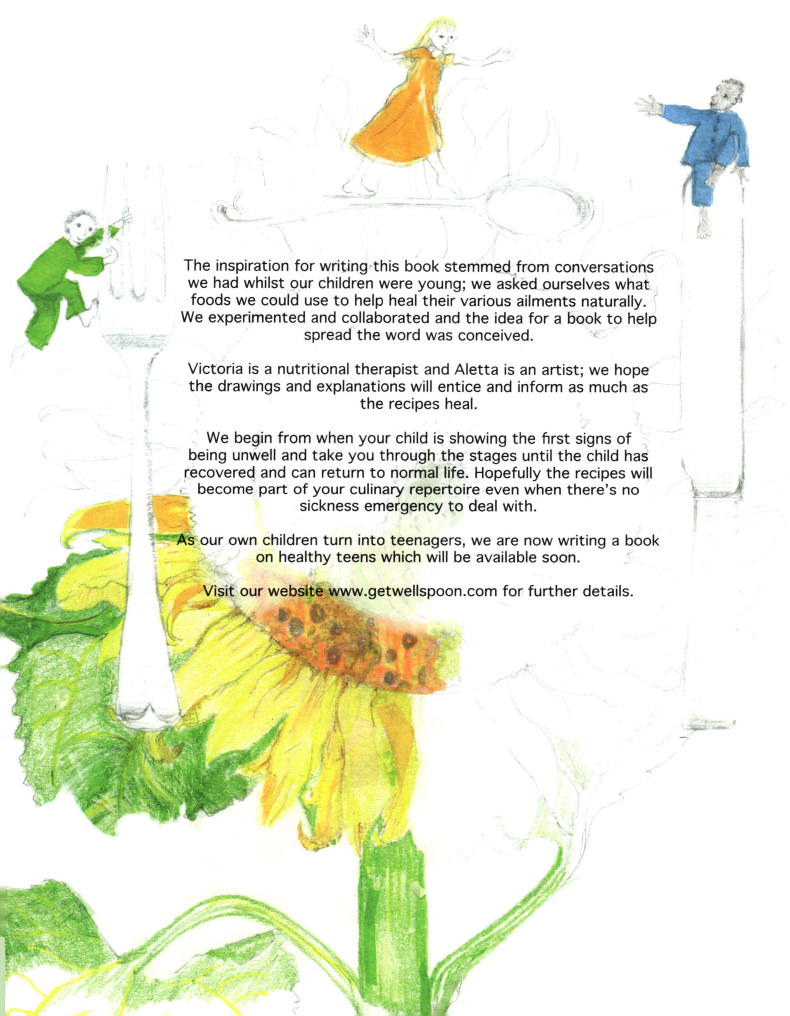

The inspiration for writing this book stemmed from conversations we had whilst our children were young; we asked ourselves what foods we could use to help heal their various ailments naturally. We experimented and collaborated and the idea for a book to help spread the word was conceived.

Victoria is a nutritional therapist and Aletta is an artist; we hope the drawings and explanations will entice and inform as much as the recipes heal.

We begin from when your child is showing the first signs of being unwell and take you through the stages until the child has recovered and can return to normal life. Hopefully the recipes will become part of your culinary repertoire even when there's no sickness emergency to deal with.

As our own children turn into teenagers, we are now writing a book on healthy teens which will be available soon.

Visit our website www.getwellspoon.com for further details.

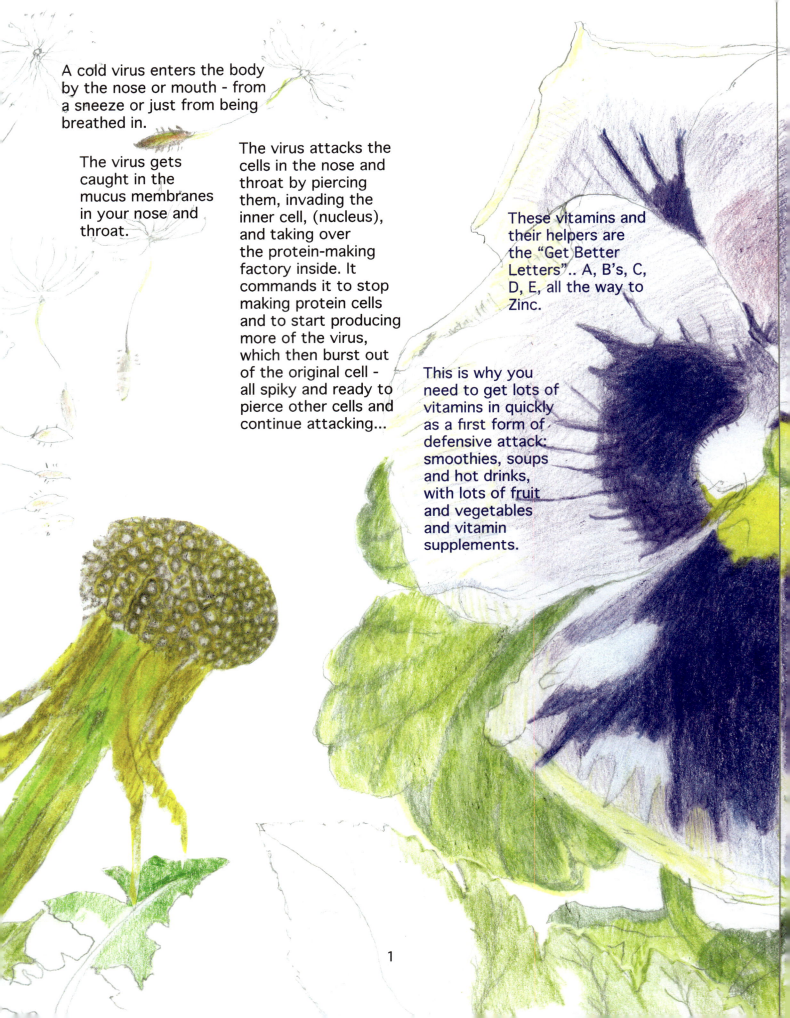

A cold virus enters the body by the nose or mouth - from a sneeze or just from being breathed in.

The virus gets caught in the mucus membranes in your nose and throat.

The virus attacks the cells in the nose and throat by piercing them, invading the inner cell, (nucleus), and taking over the protein-making factory inside. It commands it to stop making protein cells and to start producing more of the virus, which then burst out of the original cell - all spiky and ready to pierce other cells and continue attacking...

These vitamins and their helpers are the "Get Better Letters".. A, B's, C, D, E, all the way to Zinc.

This is why you need to get lots of vitamins in quickly as a first form of defensive attack: smoothies, soups and hot drinks, with lots of fruit and vegetables and vitamin supplements.

1

You get a scratchy throat or sniffy nose, and you know that you are coming down with something....

This is because all the activity in your mucus membranes produces more mucus, plus your nasal passages are getting inflamed.

Immune cells are sent out to kill the invaders.

Your body immediately sends antioxidants to the cells, to disarm the virus and the free radicals. This is the "antioxidance".

Sugar stops the immune cells from killing bacteria and it feeds the bad guys in your gut. Your body has to produce insulin to control sugar levels which uses resources and detracts from defending your body.

If you go to bed with a hot drink, lots of vitamins and keep rested and warm, your body will be able to use its resources for getting better.

This is why fizzy or sugary drinks are not a good idea to have when you are ill!

IF YOU WAKE UP FEELING WELL, THE FIGHT IS WON.

If you wake up feeling the same or worse, your body needs more support until it can fight off the virus or bacteria.

I thank my parents, Midge and David Kell, for their foodie enthusiasms, family meals and love of a feast. Not a food fashion escaped my childhood home, which resonated with the whiff of food cooking and the clatter of mealtimes. A rousing cheer for James, Ted and Boo, for more than a decade of testing and tasting. Not everything that left my kitchen was palatable, I am sorry about that soup. Thank you to my friends and family for all their encouragement. I have read hundreds of cookery books, and thousands of recipes, and am grateful for all, most especially Deborah Jarvis's "Kitchen Wizard", and Nanette Newman's "The Fun Food Factory". VK

The illustrations in this book are dedicated to my father, Bruce Ritchie, in memory of his love of botany and his joyful zest for learning and discovery. I am ever thankful to Nancy, Corinna, Joe, Iona and Oran; to the Lynch, Ritchie, Dakin and Tai families for their love and support; to Claudia for her valuable editorial input and to my wonderful friends for their kindness and encouragement. I am also grateful for the amazing resources of Kew Gardens, RHS Wisley and Chelsea Physic Garden which are vital sources of inspiration. AR

Together we would like to thank these people who generously gave us their advice and guidance when creating this book: Sally Bessada, Moira Bogue, Charlie Dossett, Michaela Eder, Annabel Freyberg, Maria Fitzjohn, Claudia Jessop, Joe Lynch, Sybil Pagnamenta, Jim Pipe, Francesca Humphrey and Eric Treuillé.

CONTENT: Victoria Kell
ILLUSTRATIONS: Aletta Ritchie
EDITORS: Claudia Jessop and Annabel Freyberg

www.getwellspoon.com

©2014

Both metric and imperial or cup measurements have been given in all recipes. Use one set of measurements only, and not a mixture of both. If you struggle to source a particular flour or sugar replacement ingredient, it is possible, though less nutritious, to use plain flour or sugar.

This book includes dishes made with nuts and nut derivatives. It is advisable for those with known allergic reactions to nuts and nut derivatives and those who may be vulnerable to these allergies to avoid dishes made with nuts or nut oils or butters.

Contents

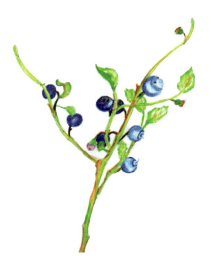

ANTHOCYANIDINS are powerful antioxidants which fight bacteria & reduce inflammation. They are found in blueberries, blackberries, black & red raspberries, strawberries, cranberries, bilberry, blackcurrant, cherry, aubergine skin, black rice & dark grapes.

Fever? Flu? What to Do

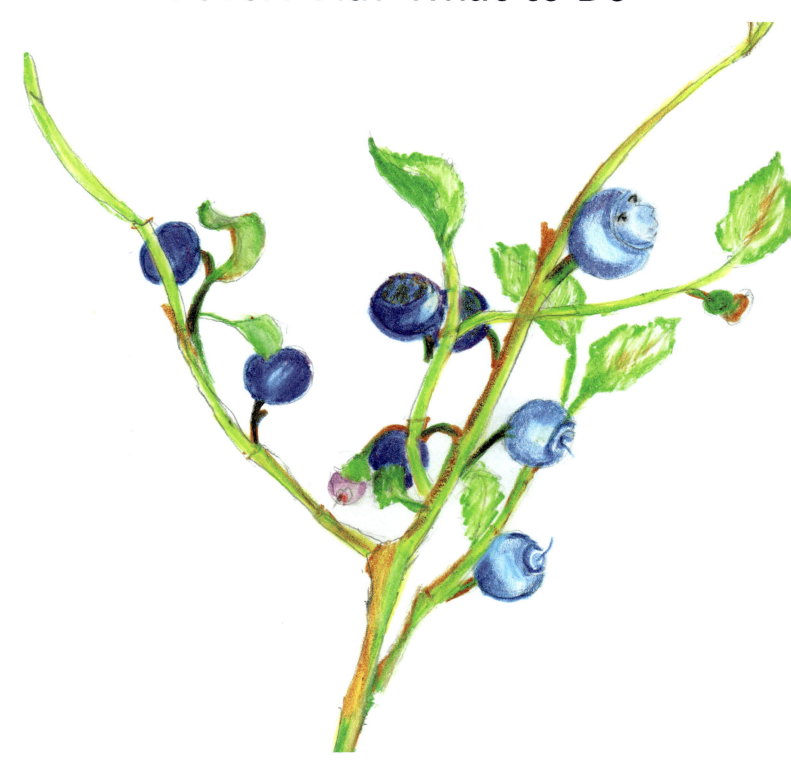

Smoothies, Hotties & Soups

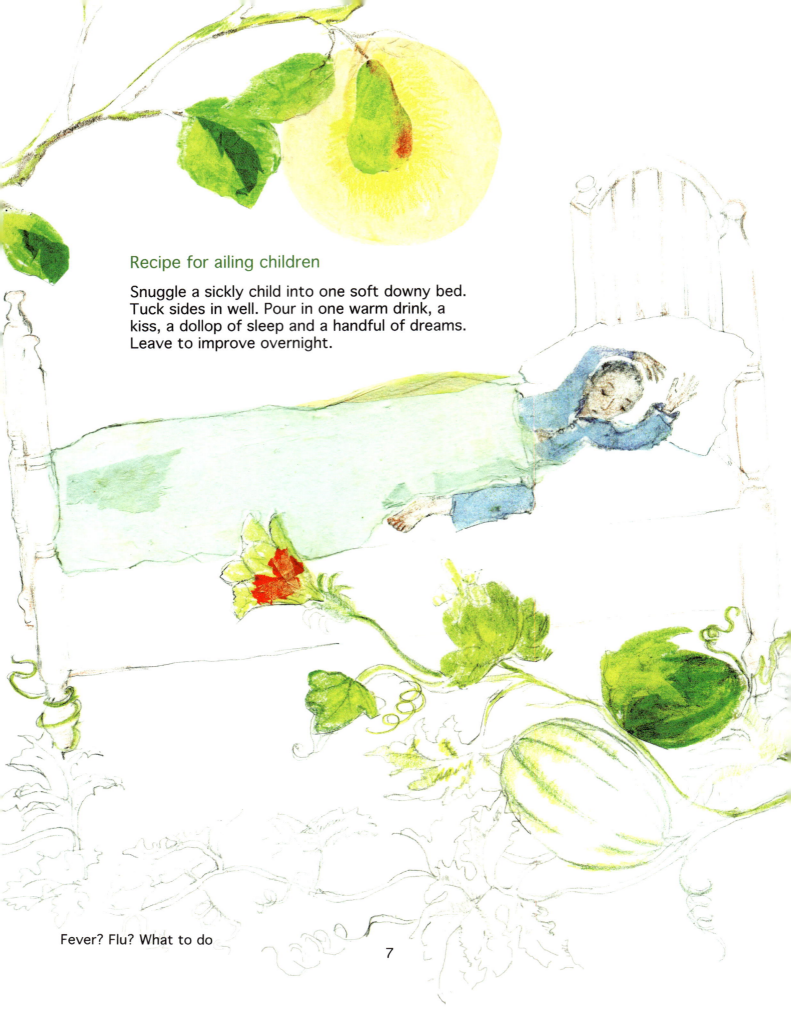

Recipe for ailing children

Snuggle a sickly child into one soft downy bed.
Tuck sides in well. Pour in one warm drink, a
kiss, a dollop of sleep and a handful of dreams.
Leave to improve overnight.

Fever? Flu? What to do

7

When your child doesn't seem well, wrap him or her up nice and warm, and either put them to bed or to snuggle up on the sofa.

Your child is unlikely to feel hungry because his or her body is about to go into battle and it doesn't want any energy dissipated, but he or she will need to keep hydrated and to take some nutrients that will help the fight.

The first thing you can give them is a smoothie, or, if your child is old enough, a hot or warm drink. A soup will also give them the nutrients they need and is easy for the body to digest, so will not be taxing. You are looking to arm the body's internal fighters with the weapons they need to fight off the invaders - the vitamins and other nutrients that are used in attack and defence. The body needs to sleep to save energy so that the battle can be fought as effectively as possible.

So snuggle them up warm, give them a drink and some soup. The recipes in this chapter will give you some simple ideas.

The reason you can give them food with strong flavours, (like garlic and ginger), is because the sense of taste and smell is weakened, partly because zinc is diverted to fight the free radicals and to support the antioxidants.

If they wake up feeling better, the white blood cells have killed off the virus and the antioxidants have disarmed the free radicals.

If they wake up and feel the same or worse, then their body needs a little more help. Look through the book for recipes to help fight fevers, flu, viruses and tummy troubles.

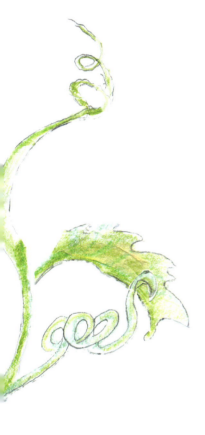

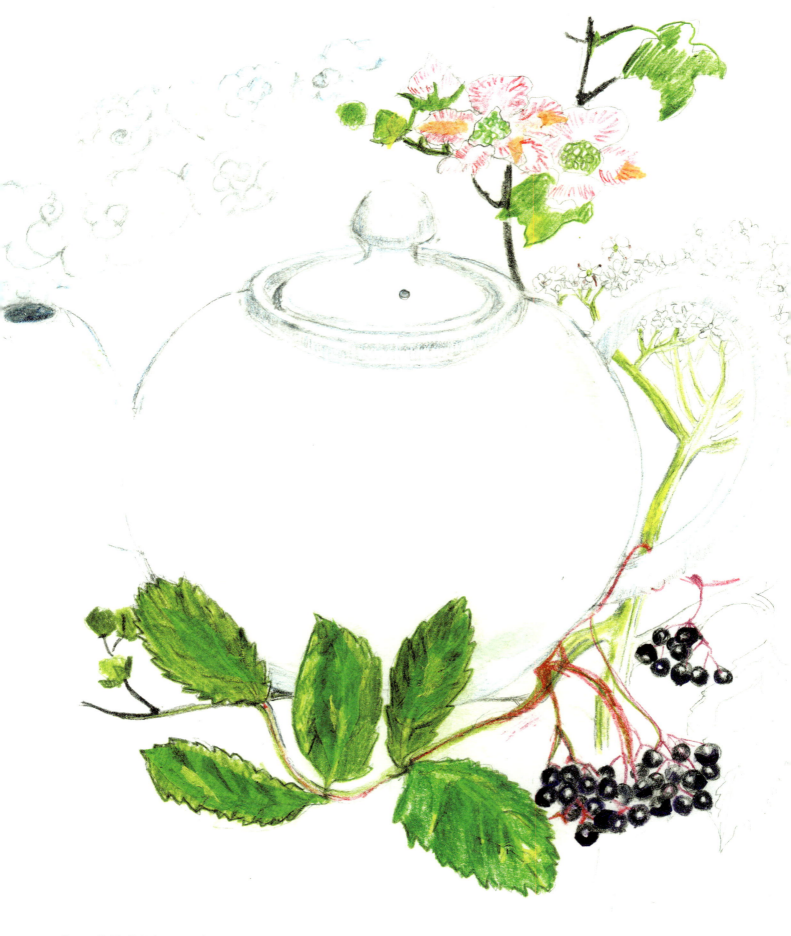

Research shows that having a warm drink fights off colds and other snotties

Buy your honey wisely. Try to get the best quality you can, and check on the label there is no added sugar. Manuka honey from New Zealand has special properties. It is antibacterial, antiviral, and antimicrobial. It is also an antioxidant, antiseptic and anti-inflammatory, the perfect sweetener for warm drinks to aid recovery.

Agave Nectar is a natural sweetener made from the blue agave plant from Mexico. You only need to use a little as it is 4 times sweeter than normal sugar, but it has a low glycemic load which means that it will not spike up blood sugar levels, which is important when you don't feel well.

Elderberry Hottie

Stir a couple of teaspoons of elderberry extract from a health food shop into warm water.

If you feel a bit off colour, tired or not hungry, these could be signs that your body is diverting its resources to fight a virus. There is a special substance in elderberry called interferon which "interferes" with the spikes of a virus (such as a cold), by covering them up so they can't attack - thus stopping the virus from getting into your body.

Ginger for a Winger

A glug of ginger cordial or fresh grated ginger with cinnamon, clove, lemon and manuka honey, steeped in hot water. Strain before serving.

Ginger is a great antibacterial and antiviral. You might get away with it even if your child doesn't normally enjoy strong tastes as, when you feel off colour, you lose your sense of taste. Ginger can calm coughing, is anti-inflammatory and soothes tummy aches. You can use fresh grated ginger infusion as a base for a fruit drink - try mixed with warm apple or orange juice.

A Wise Drink for a Sore Throat

Use fresh sage if you have it, and leave to steep in hot water for a few minutes. Remove leaves before serving, and sweeten with manuka honey.

Granny's Hot St Clements & Honey

Warm up some orange juice and add a teaspoon of honey, or squeeze juice of 1 lemon into a cup, and pour on hot water.

Other Teas

Mint tea can help stomach pains and is an invigorating tonic. Rosehip and Hibiscus teas are a lovely pink colour, and are full of vitamin C. Camomile tea will calm emotionally and can help to soothe inflamed membranes which is useful if you have a cold.

Use tea bags or loose tea and sweeten with honey or agave syrup.

Soothie Smoothies for a Spiky Throat

When you have a glut of fruit, put some in the freezer, and it can be used in drinks. Regard it as a store-cupboard essential. Using frozen fruit also keeps the drinks chilled, which can be soothing.

Tropical Throat Soother

Peel, chop and blend 1 ripe mango, 2 ripe peaches and 1 ripe banana. Add 100ml (½ cup) of coconut milk to get a pleasant consistency. The mango, peaches and banana can be frozen and used from the freezer.

Banana skin goes black when it is frozen but the banana inside is still good. If you beat it till it is smooth, it is like ice-cream.

This is high in antioxidants, beta carotene, cryptoxanthin and vitamin C. Also the potassium, fibre, fructooligosaccharides (FOS) and short chain fatty acids will support the body's immune-attacking system and healthy gut. Bananas contain tryptophan which the body converts to serotonin, a good mood hormone.

Berry Good for You

Whizz frozen berries (strawberries, blueberries, blackberries) and a banana with vanilla rice milk or almond milk for a delicious pink drink!

Strawberries are natural painkillers, and have fantastic antioxidant qualities. Like blueberries, they contain anthocyanins which are linked to good eyesight. Bananas have fructooligosaccharides which support the tummy, and rice milk contains B vitamins.

Watermelon Heaven

Blend watermelon flesh and seeds with some ice for a cool refreshing drink.

Watermelons are hydrating and cleansing, and are thought to soothe feverish thirst.

The carotenoids and vitamin C in the melon are used for the defence system and lungs whilst the seeds contain lots of zinc, brilliant for growth and immunity.

Fever? Flu? What to do

Feeling Peaky Drinks & Soups

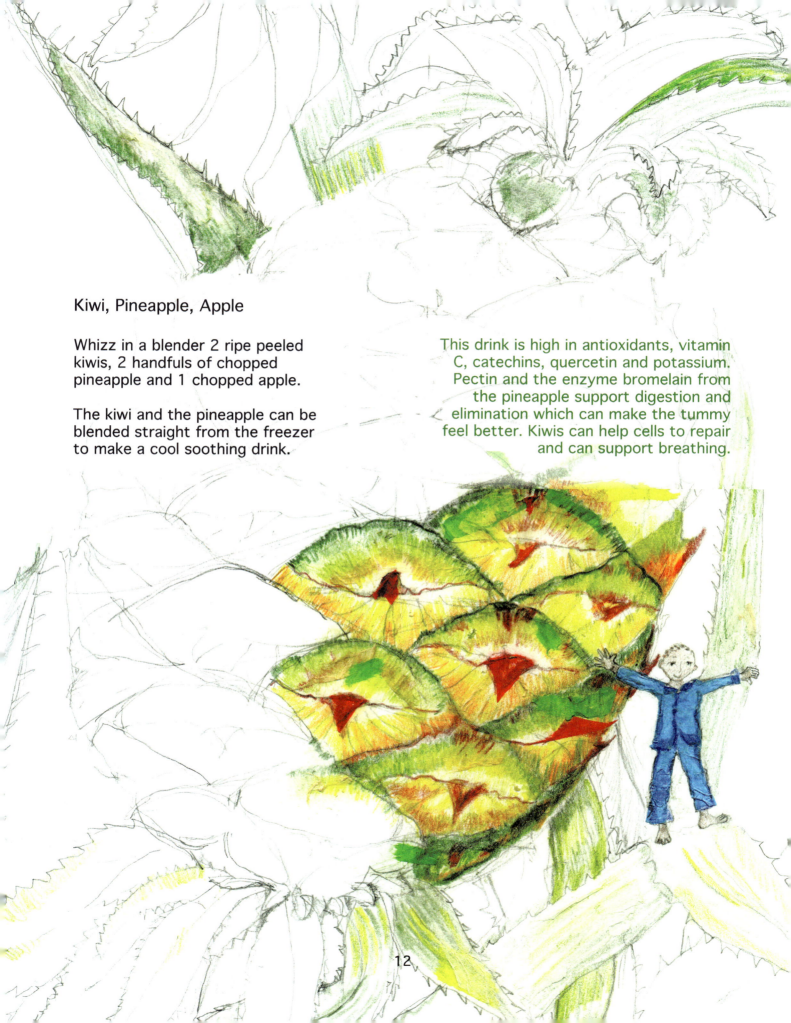

Kiwi, Pineapple, Apple

Whizz in a blender 2 ripe peeled kiwis, 2 handfuls of chopped pineapple and 1 chopped apple.

The kiwi and the pineapple can be blended straight from the freezer to make a cool soothing drink.

This drink is high in antioxidants, vitamin C, catechins, quercetin and potassium. Pectin and the enzyme bromelain from the pineapple support digestion and elimination which can make the tummy feel better. Kiwis can help cells to repair and can support breathing.

Soups for Colds & Sniffles

Leek & Ginger Soup

3 leeks, washed, trimmed & sliced
½ tablespoon fresh grated ginger
olive oil for cooking
500ml (2 cups) vegetable stock

In a saucepan, lightly sweat the leeks in olive oil until soft. Add the ginger. Cover with vegetable stock and simmer for 15 minutes. Pour into a blender and blend until smooth. Add more water if needed for a soupy consistency.

This lovely soup helps to clear up phlegm.

Brown Onion & Mushroom Soup

1kg (2lb) onions, red or brown, sliced
2 handfuls mushrooms, finely chopped
1 tablespoon olive oil
1 litre (4 cups) vegetable stock
2 cloves garlic, crushed
juice of 1 lemon
handful chopped parsley & chives

In a saucepan, lightly sweat the onion and mushrooms in olive oil until golden. Cover with vegetable stock, add garlic and lemon juice, bring to the boil and then simmer for 15 minutes. Add the parsley and chives. Whizz in a blender for a smooth consistency if preferred.

This soup is especially good for helping to fight shivery colds, blocked noses and congested sinuses.

Like garlic and leeks, onions help clear the respiratory system and have antiseptic qualities, and mushrooms contain a valuable antioxidant called L-ergothioneine and are full of potassium.

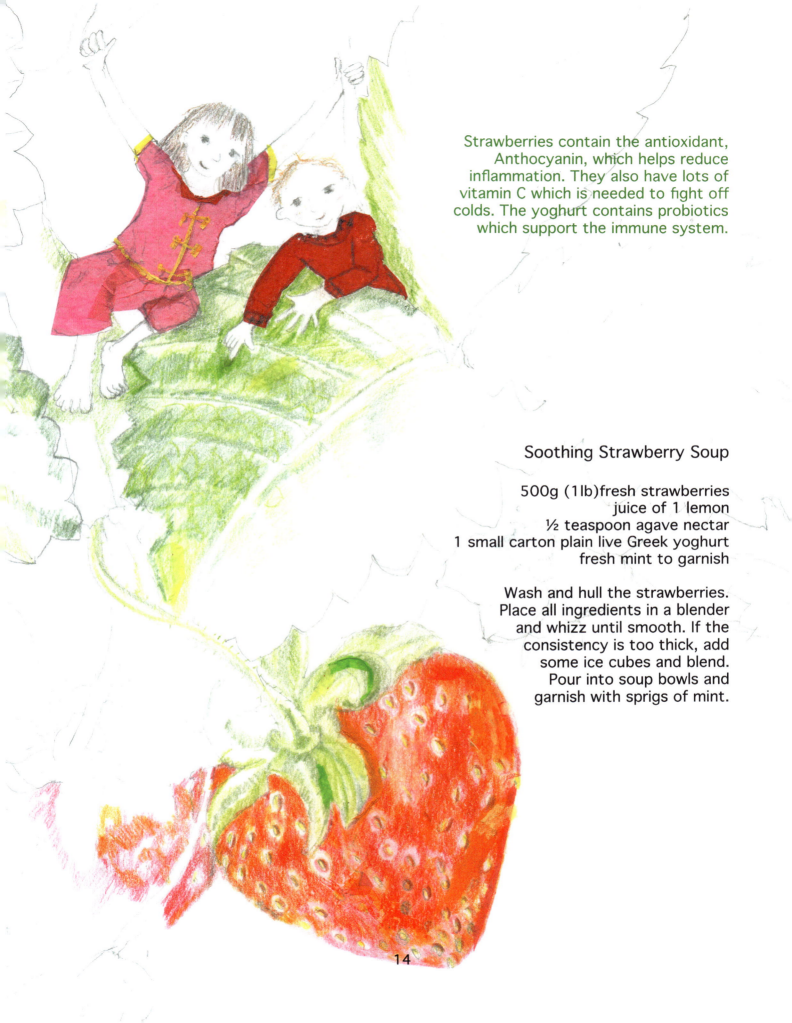

Strawberries contain the antioxidant, Anthocyanin, which helps reduce inflammation. They also have lots of vitamin C which is needed to fight off colds. The yoghurt contains probiotics which support the immune system.

Soothing Strawberry Soup

500g (1lb) fresh strawberries
juice of 1 lemon
½ teaspoon agave nectar
1 small carton plain live Greek yoghurt
fresh mint to garnish

Wash and hull the strawberries. Place all ingredients in a blender and whizz until smooth. If the consistency is too thick, add some ice cubes and blend. Pour into soup bowls and garnish with sprigs of mint.

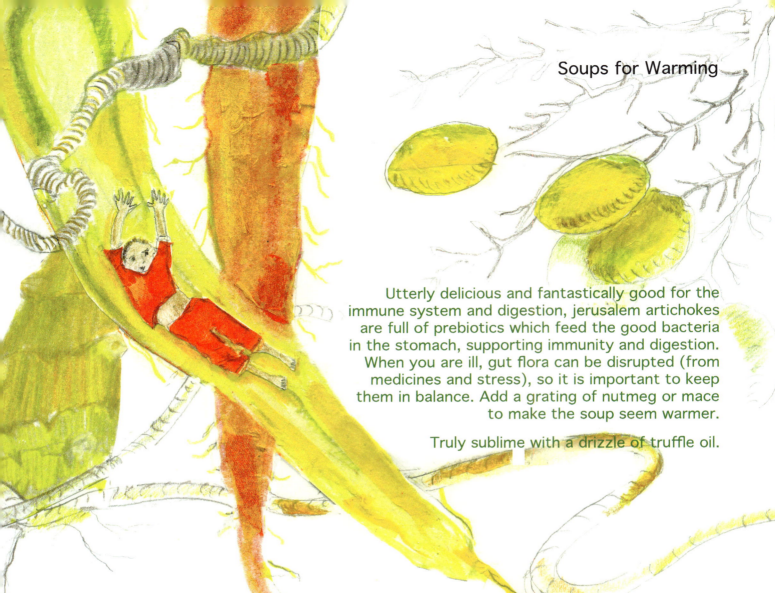

Utterly delicious and fantastically good for the
immune system and digestion, jerusalem artichokes
are full of prebiotics which feed the good bacteria
in the stomach, supporting immunity and digestion.
When you are ill, gut flora can be disrupted (from
medicines and stress), so it is important to keep
them in balance. Add a grating of nutmeg or mace
to make the soup seem warmer.

Truly sublime with a drizzle of truffle oil.

Jerusalem Artichoke Soup

500g (1lb) jerusalem artichokes, chopped
½ sweet potato, cubed
1 onion, chopped
500ml (2 cups) vegetable stock

In a saucepan, lightly sweat the vegetables in olive oil until soft.
Cover with vegetable stock and simmer for 15 minutes or until the artichoke is soft.
Pour into a blender and blend until smooth, adding more water if necessary for a soupy consistency.
The sweet potato is partly to add colour otherwise this soup is quite grey.
You could replace the potato with beetroot for a pink soup.

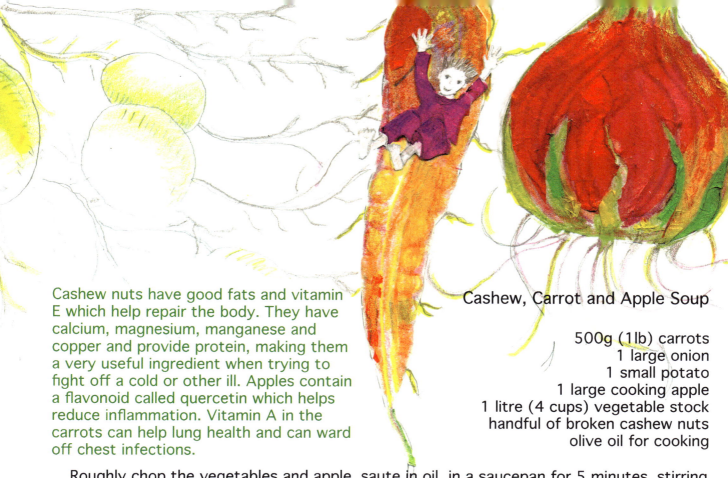

Cashew nuts have good fats and vitamin E which help repair the body. They have calcium, magnesium, manganese and copper and provide protein, making them a very useful ingredient when trying to fight off a cold or other ill. Apples contain a flavonoid called quercetin which helps reduce inflammation. Vitamin A in the carrots can help lung health and can ward off chest infections.

Cashew, Carrot and Apple Soup

500g (1lb) carrots
1 large onion
1 small potato
1 large cooking apple
1 litre (4 cups) vegetable stock
handful of broken cashew nuts
olive oil for cooking

Roughly chop the vegetables and apple, saute in oil in a saucepan for 5 minutes, stirring occasionally. Add the remaining ingredients, bring to the boil and simmer for 30 minutes until the vegetables are just tender. Cool a little before blending to a suitable consistency.

Sweet Potato, Squash and Ginger Soup

1 sweet potato, cubed
1 butternut squash, cubed
1 onion, chopped
2 cloves garlic, finely squished
2cm ginger, finely sliced
1 handful split red lentils, washed
500ml (2 cups) vegetable stock
or 1 tin of coconut milk & 1 tin of water

Sweat the vegetables in a saucepan until soft. Cover with vegetable stock, or coconut milk and water, and add lentils. Pour into a blender and blend until smooth.

The beta carotene in the butternut squash and sweet potato provides antioxidant support to fight free radicals produced by a virus or bacteria attacking the body. Sweet potatoes also have lots of vitamin C and E which protect the immune system.

Garlic, onion and ginger are antiviral and antibacterial and provide immune support. Lentils provide B vitamins which support the antioxidants. All provide easily digestible fibre which means the body will not have to work too hard to digest and release the nutrients. The addition of coconut milk will provide caprylic acid which will support the health of the gut - useful if medicines are being taken.

Soups for Colds and Sniffles

Chicken soup has been medically proven to reduce cold symptoms

Chicken Soup

1 medium sized organic chicken
1 pack of chicken wings
3 large onions
1 large sweet potato
3 parsnips
2 turnips
12 large carrots
6 celery stems
1 bunch of parsley

Clean the chicken, put it in a large pot and cover with water. Bring the water to boil. Add the chicken wings, onions, sweet potato, parsnips, turnips and carrots. Simmer for about 1½ hours. Scoop off the fat from the surface as it accumulates.

Add the parsley and celery. Keep simmering for another 45 minutes. Remove the chicken. The chicken is not used further for the soup, (though pieces can be added when the child is feeling better, if they want a more robust meal). Whizz in blender and add water for consistency.

This recipe makes a large amount of soup. It will last a couple of days, or you can freeze a batch. It is scientifically proven[1] to reduce the symptoms of a cold.

[1] University of Nebraska Medical Centre, 2008

Up the ante by adding some mushrooms as they contain lentinan. Lentinan has been shown to be even more effective than prescription drugs against influenza and other viruses. Mushrooms also contain a powerful antioxidant called L-ergothioneine.

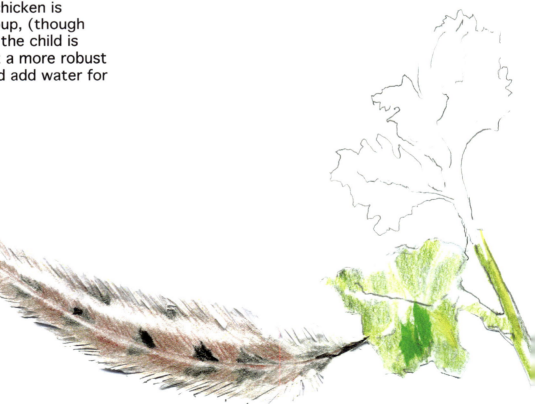

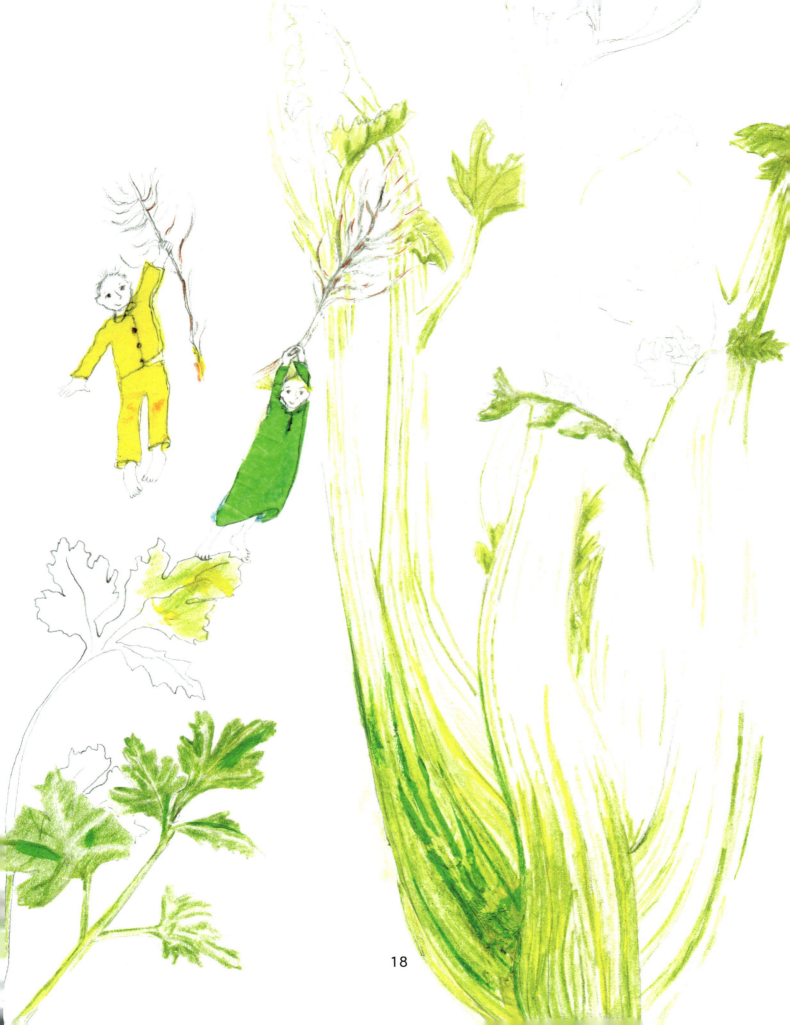

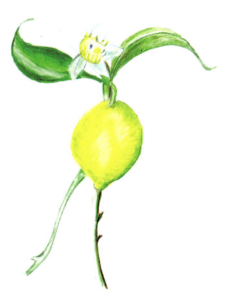

HESPERIDIN is the flavonoid found in lots of citrus fruits like oranges, tangerines, grapefruits, clementines, lemons, limes, mandarins, pomelos, kumquats, ugli fruits & tangelos. It is an antioxidant, anti-inflammatory & a natural sedative.

ALLIUMS are the onion & garlic family. They contain an organosulfide which fights bacteria & micro-organisms with its sulphur containing enzymes. Organosulphurs are powerful antioxidants who scavenge free radicals, stop fats from going bad & stop inflammatory messengers inside the body.

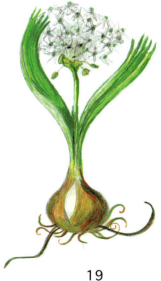

Fighting Chills & Other ills

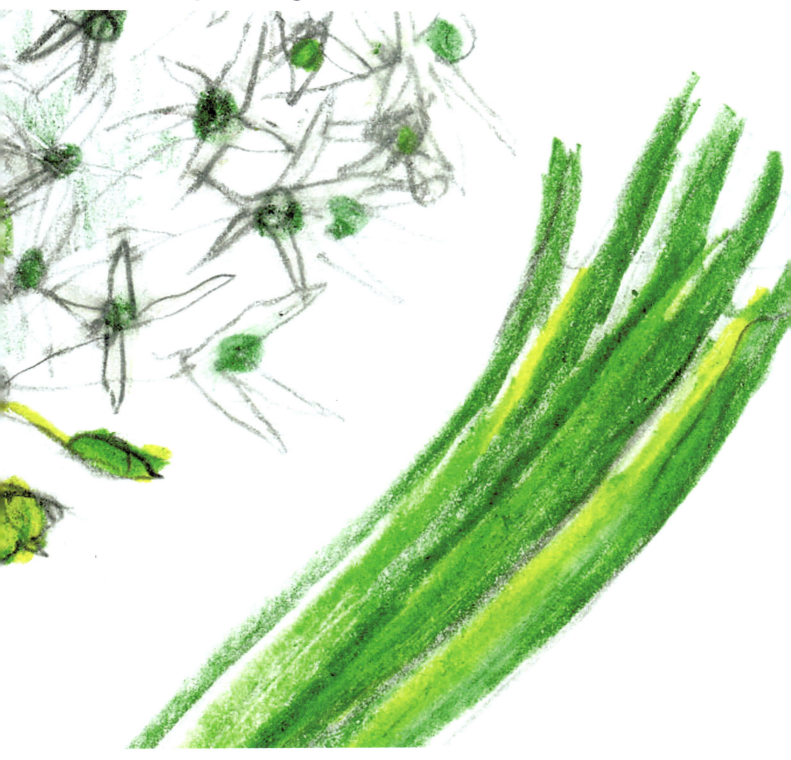

Recipes to Ease Sore Throats, Chicken Pox & Colds

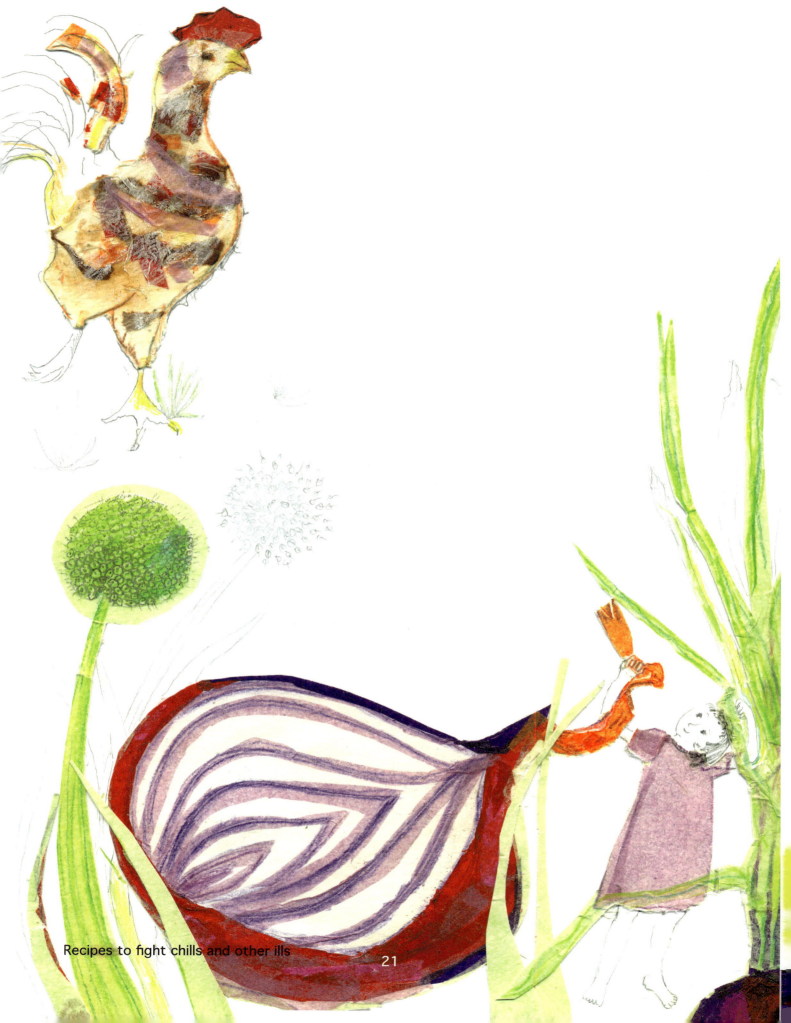

Recipes to fight chills and other ills

21

Fox the Chicken Pox

1 chicken thigh per person
1 onion, finely sliced
3 cloves garlic, crushed
1 large carrot, finely chopped
shiitake mushrooms - a generous handful (if dried, soak before using)
500ml (2 cups) stock
220g (1¼ cups) quinoa grains
olive oil for cooking

Brown the chicken thighs, with the skin on, in a small amount of olive oil. Remove the chicken and add onion and carrot to the pan. Cook until onion turns golden and add the mushrooms and garlic. Add chicken and stock. Add quinoa, bring to the boil and simmer for 20 minutes, until the quinoa is cooked and opened up. Remove the chicken skin and bones before you serve.

Superfood quinoa is a complete, easily digestible protein and complex carbohydrate. The complex carbohydrate qualities help to regulate blood sugar which supports the immune system, thus aiding recovery. It has plenty of the amino acid, Lysine, which is essential for tissue growth and repair. Chicken has protein, healing enzymes, B vitamins and minerals. Onions, garlic and shiitake mushrooms are effective virus fighters.

Play calamine lotion "dot-the-dots". Scabs are part of the fighting process; they protect the body from outside germs. They are made of yucky dead stuff - dead blood cells, skin cells, pus and other stuff your body has chucked out. Don't be tempted to "pick and eat", make a fuss about the pus.

Weasle the Sneazle Measles Broth

To fight off bacterial infection, this comforting and super nutritious stew is easy to eat and to digest.

2 onions, finely sliced
2 cloves garlic, finely sliced
thumb-sized piece ginger, finely sliced
root veg, peeled, chopped into 2cm pieces:
1 large sweet potato
2 potatoes
2 carrots
1 parsnip
turnip or swede, celeriac etc (as liked)
vegetable stock
wine vinegar or slices of lemon
large handful red lentils
1 organic salmon steak per person
generous handful flat leaf parsley to garnish

Fry onions in the bottom of a heavy saucepan until golden.
Add the root vegetables, garlic and ginger and lightly cook, then add enough hot water with bouillon or vegetable stock to cover plus two fingers width. Add lentils, turn down heat and cook for 20 to 30 minutes.
Wrap the salmon in foil, squirt with wine vinegar spray or garnish with lemon. Add a tiny bit of olive oil, wrap up and cook at 180C (350F/Gas 4) in the oven for 20 minutes.

Place vegetable and lentil stew in the bottom of a bowl and place the salmon on top.
Garnish with parsley.

This is choc-a-bloc with antioxidants, vitamins and carotenes from the vegetables, and digestible fibre to keep the gut moving. There are powerful antiviral and antibacterial agents in the onion, garlic and ginger, while red lentils are full of B vitamins which help fight infections and keep energy levels up, as well as soluble fibre to keep blood sugar in check. Finally, the fish provides lots of protein to build you up, essential fats to reduce inflammation and minerals that help fight infections. Parsley gives antioxidant protection, helps kidney function and is a source of calcium.

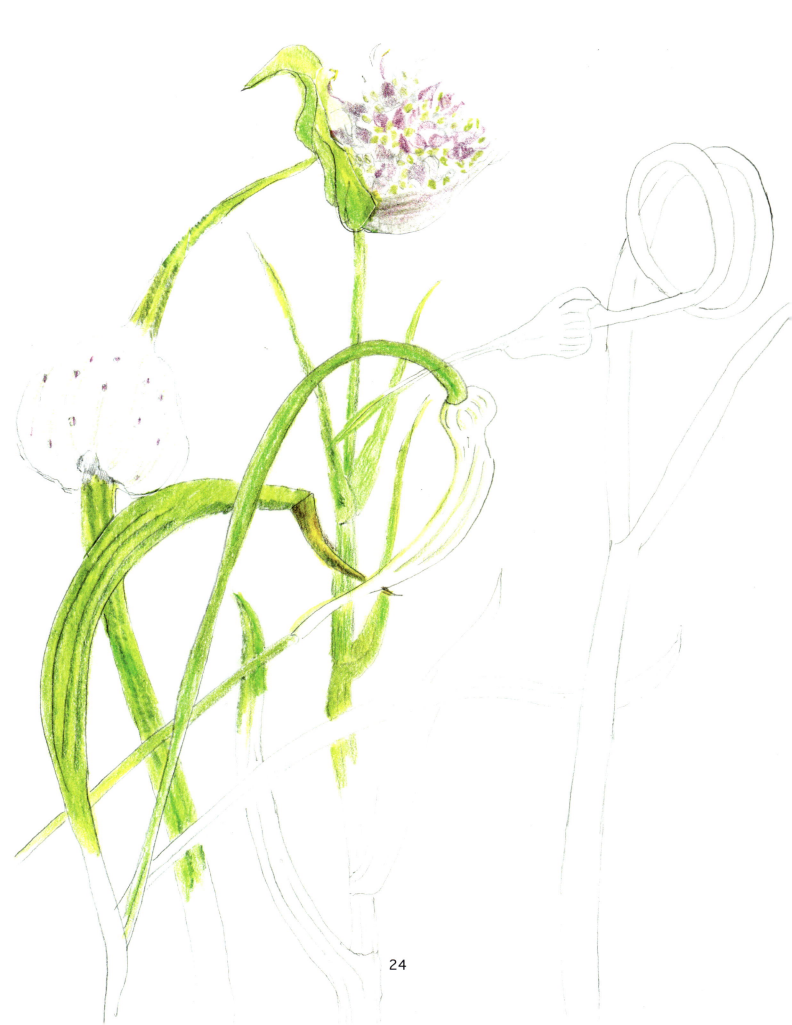

Let Them Eat Immuni-cake

12 grated carrots
2 tablespoons manuka honey
220g (1¼ cups) raisins
4 eggs
125ml (½ cup) coconut or vegetable oil
2 apples stewed to apple sauce
2 teaspoons vanilla extract
220g (⅔ cup) crushed pineapple, drained
680g (5½ cups) mixed wheat-free flour (quinoa/barley/millet)
1 ½ teaspoons baking soda
small pinch salt
4 teaspoons ground cinnamon
220g (1¾ cups) chopped walnuts

In a medium bowl, combine grated carrots, raisins and honey. Set aside for 60 minutes.
Preheat oven to 180C (350F/Gas 4). Grease and flour two 9-inch cake tins, or muffin tin.
In a large bowl, beat eggs until light. Gradually beat in the apple sauce, oil and vanilla.
Stir in the pineapple. Combine the flour, baking soda, salt and cinnamon; stir into the wet
mixture until absorbed. Finally, stir in the carrot mixture and the walnuts. Pour evenly into
the prepared tins.
Bake for 45 to 50 minutes in the oven, until the cake is baked, (test with a skewer or
sharp knife). Cool for 10 minutes before removing from tin. If making muffins, bake for 40
minutes or until they are cooked.

When appetite is low, this cake is a great way of getting in some vegetables, protein, nuts
and fruit. Cinnamon is highly antioxidant and considered antimicrobial. Apples, coconut
oil and pineapple support digestion, and pineapples are also full of manganese which is an
essential component of the antioxidant defence, and the CCS and CCZ compounds which
boost immunity.

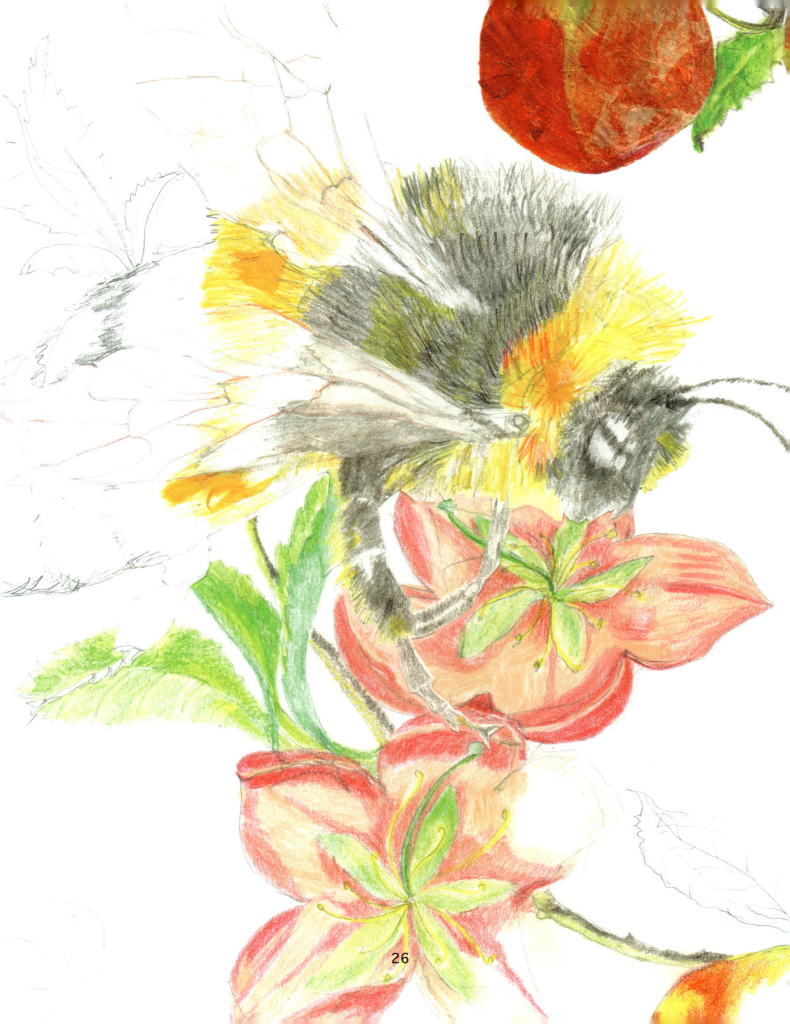

Raspberry Cool

220g (8oz) raspberries
220g (¾ cup) probiotic Greek yogurt
1 ripe banana
2 teaspoons manuka honey

Whizz all ingredients except honey in a blender. Then, slightly warm the honey, and drizzle over the top of the fool so that it melts in. Chill in the fridge.

The ellagic acid in raspberries is a powerful antioxidant and the phytonutrients called quercetin and anthocyanins, (which give raspberries their fabulous colour), are also powerful protectors. The probiotic yogurt and banana help to keep gut bacteria healthy, (which supports immunity), and manuka honey has properties which help fight off infections, bacterial or viral.

Honey & Lemon Jelly Wobbles

1 ½ tablespoons lemon juice
2 tablespoons lemon verbena tea
2 tablespoons manuka honey
2 tablespoons powdered gelatin or seaweed equivalent
sugar substitute (eg. xylitol)

Put lemon juice, water and honey in a heat-resistant bowl and mix well. Sprinkle the gelatin in and soak for around 15 minutes. Make a bain-marie to heat the mixture and melt the gelatin in. Pour into ice-cube or other moulds and cool in the fridge for two hours. Take jellies out of moulds and roll in sugar substitute.

Silky and soothing, these wibbly balls will soothe a sore throat. Lemon verbena is anti-spasmodic and de-stressing. It is also an expectorant and eases colds and fevers.

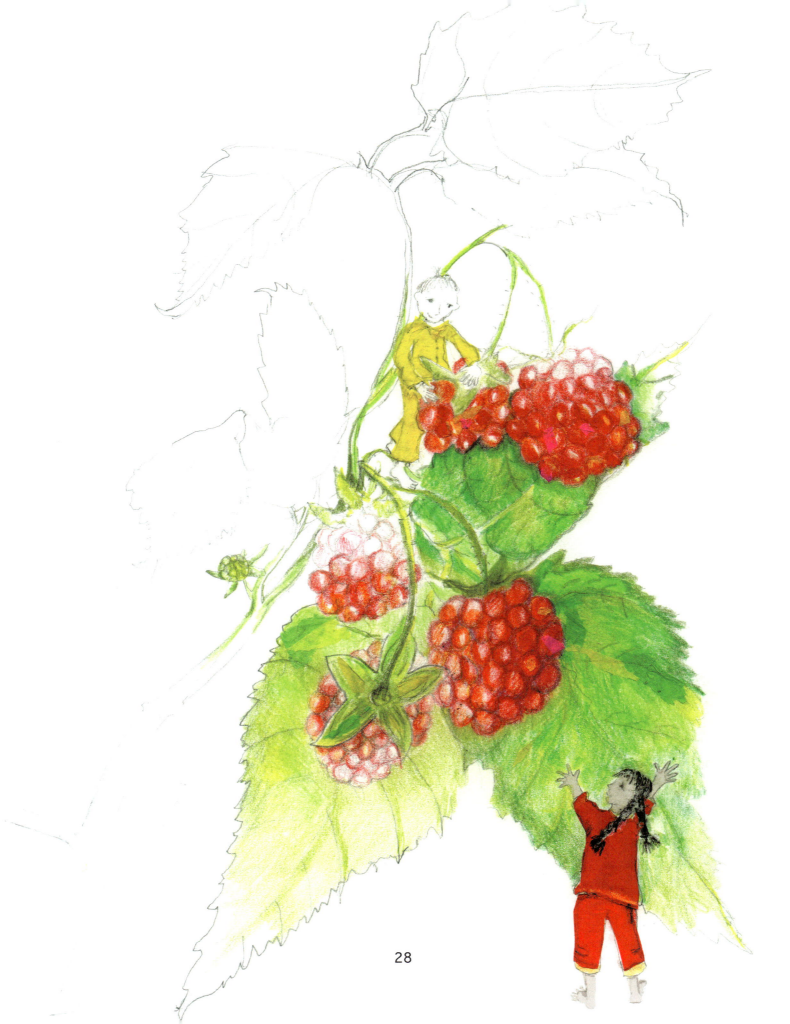

Stoat in the Throat?

It can be difficult to swallow with a stoat in your throat. These treats help soothe sore or scratchy throats.

Avocado & Banana Crush Creme

Whizz a frozen banana and a ripe avocado in a blender. Eat immediately before it discolours, or squeeze lemon or lime juice over to prevent it from turning brown.

Avocados are full of vitamin E and good fats, whilst bananas are full of potassium and prebiotics; together they make a cooling soothing concoction of goodness.

Raspberry Sweets

Freeze raspberries and suck slowly to soothe swollen sore throats. Grapes, blueberries or blackberries can be used as well. Cut the fruit in half or smaller as the sweet needs to be small to avoid the child choking, or being too cold for a little mouth.

Silky Strawberry Soother

1 punnet of frozen strawberries, green stalks taken off, whizzed in a blender with
1 packet (275g/9oz) of silken tofu and its liquid and
2 tablespoons of clear honey or apple juice to sweeten.

This will be icy and thick. Serve at once

Pomegranate Sorbet

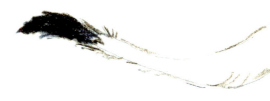

Freeze pomegranate juice, break into rough chunks and whizz in a blender to a sorbet consistency

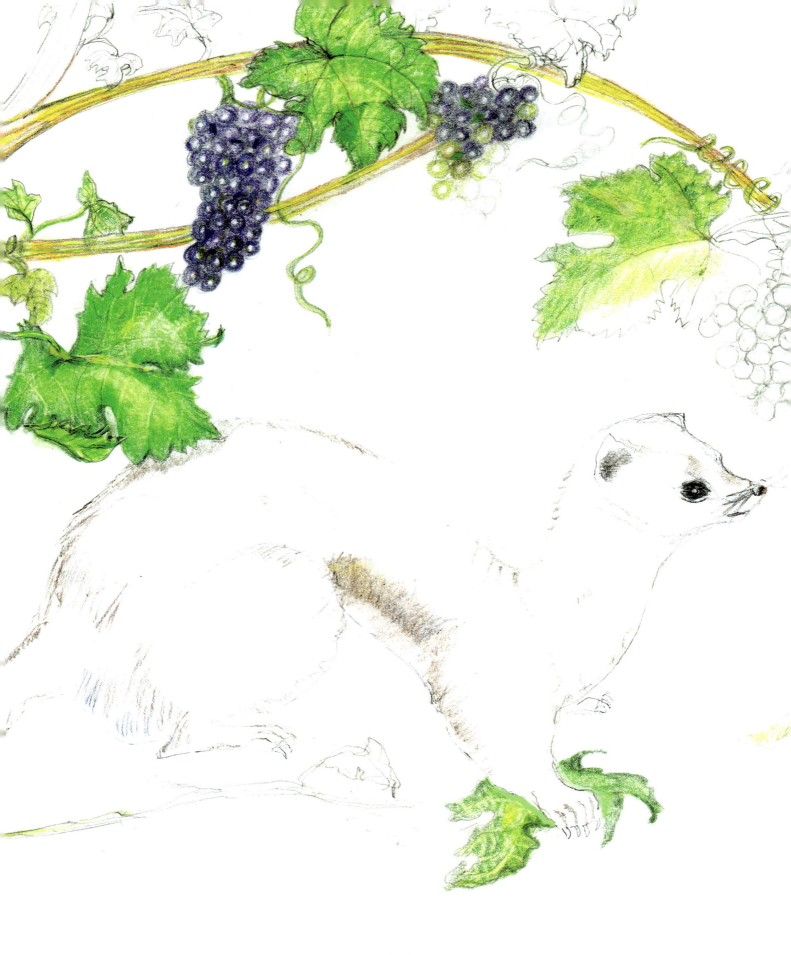

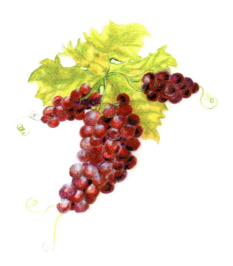

PROANTHOCYANIDIN is a group of flavonols found in grape seeds & grape skin, cocoa beans, apple, cinnamon, bilberry, cranberry, blackcurrant, green & black tea. This antioxidant protects collagen & elastin - two proteins found in connective tissue, useful if you have problems with joints, skin, muscles & blood vessels.

QUERCETIN is an anti-inflammatory & antioxidant flavonoid, it often stores vitamin C. It is found in apple, citrus fruit, buckwheat, onion (especially red), tea, berries (cherry, raspberry & cranberry), tomatoes, red grapes, broccoli, green leafy vegetables, honey from eucalyptus, capers & lovage. Quercetin helps with respiratory problems & may be a slight anti-depressant.

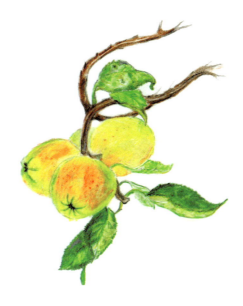

The Tummy Wars

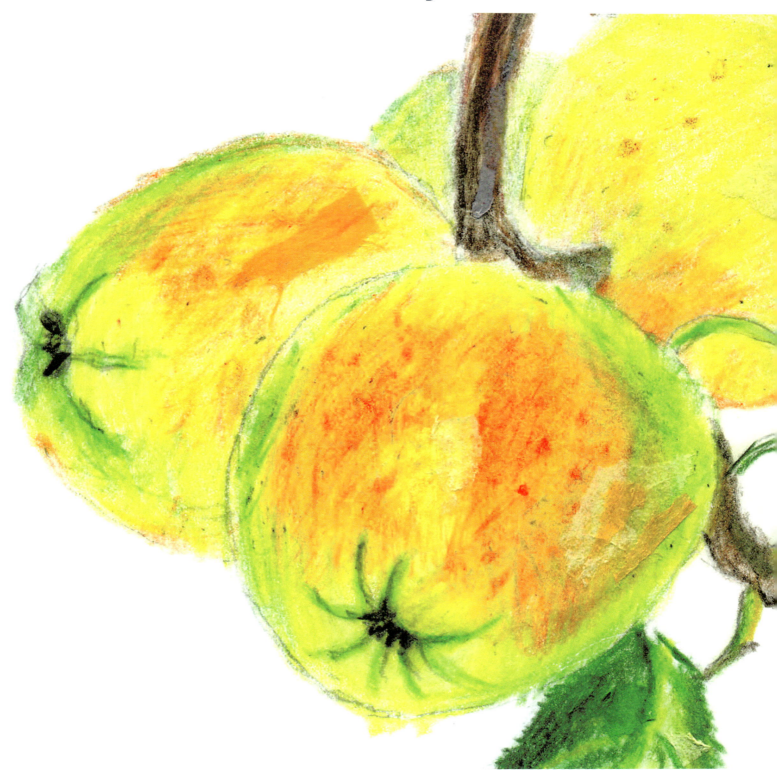

Recipes to Help Constipation

Recipes for constipation, diarrhoea & to build good gut bacteria

When your child is suffering from constipation, it is crucial to get things "moving" again and to keep hydrated so that it isn't painful to pass a stool. It is healthy to pass a stool at least twice a day. If your child has not passed a stool in a day, then try to give a little nutritional help - bowel movements can be affected by a change in environment, (such as travel or different food), stress and dehydration.

When children are suffering from diarrhoea, it is important to rehydrate as so much liquid has been lost, and to regulate stool movement. Generally they have diarrhoea because they have a bug that the body is trying to evacuate, so it is a good idea to let it run its course, as much as possible, as long as they can keep hydration up and stay at home.

Whether they are constipated or have diarrhoea, they won't feel like eating, so don't worry if appetites are small.

There are some foods and spices that have the dual effect of either slowing down digestion or stimulating digestion depending on what your body needs - very useful! Apples and pears are great for tummy problems as they have soluble fibre which stimulates bowel movement if you are constipated and slows things down if you have diarrhoea - it regulates peristalsis, which is the involuntary undulating muscle movement of the gut, which moves food from your stomach to your bottom.

Apple juice and pear juice would be great drinks to start off with. Depending on the weather, add warm water if you need something warm and comforting or ice to make it cool and refreshing.

Camomile has a faint apple taste, so a mix of weak camomile tea and apple juice would be lovely. Camomile is also very soothing for the tummy.

Cinnamon also speeds or slows digestion depending on what you need; try a warm apple drink with a sprinkle of cinnamon.

These two unusual drinks also help to regulate bowel movement:

Fennel seed tea; infuse half a teaspoon of whole fennel seeds in boiling water for five minutes.

Rose tea; steep a couple of fresh fragrant red rose petals (or dried ones, available from herbalists), with the white core cut off, in boiling water for a few minutes.

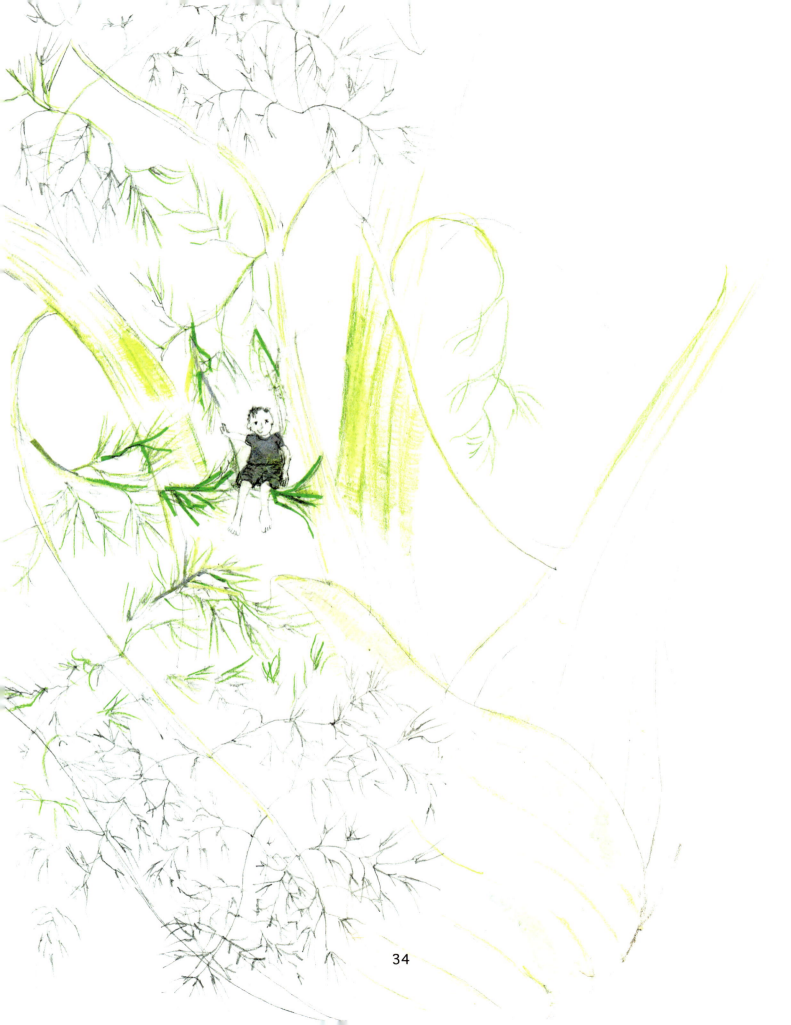

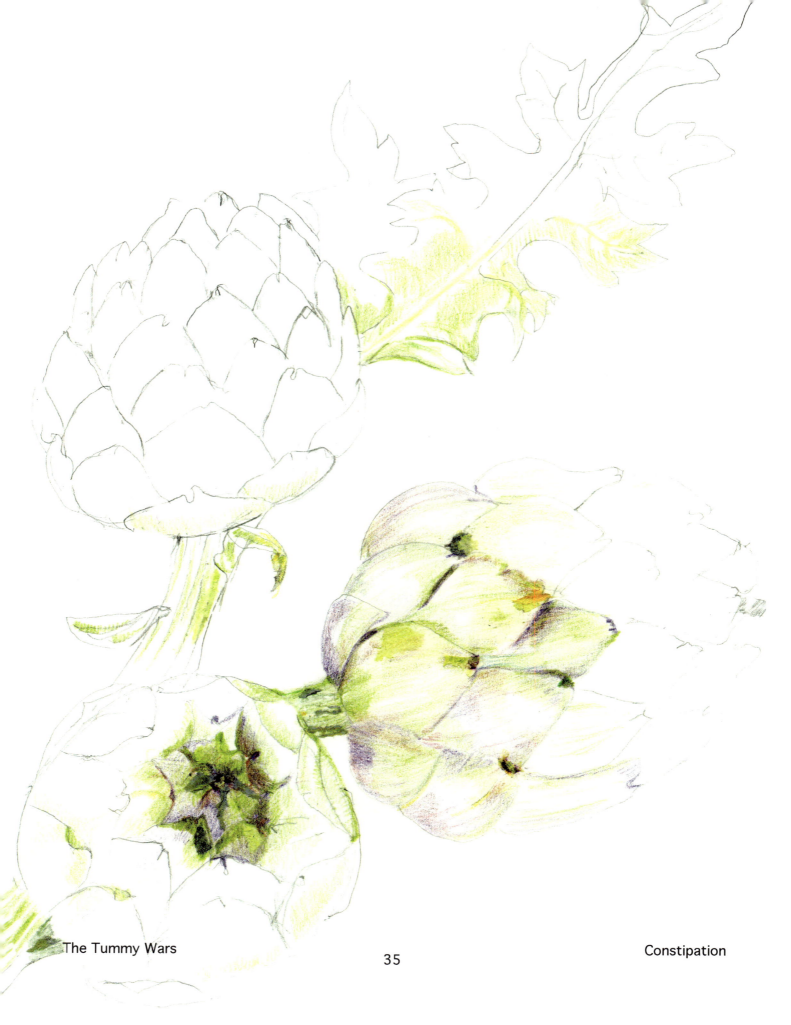

Globe artichokes - baby ones or hearts - are very useful to get things moving again. Whizz into a dip, or stew in olive oil in a covered pan until tender.

Artichoke Rice

6 baby artichokes or artichoke hearts
220g (1¼ cups) long grain brown rice
juice of 1 lemon
2 garlic cloves, chopped
2 tablespoons olive oil
1 teaspoon butter (optional)

Cut up the artichoke into small pieces and sprinkle lemon juice over them. Fry in oil in a saucepan with the rice and garlic, then add a pint (500ml/2 cups) of water; allow to cook very gently for about 45 minutes with the lid on the pan. Stir in a teaspoon of butter before serving if you wish.

Artichokes nourish the good bacteria in the gut by providing fructooligosaccharides, a sugar that the good bacteria like to feed on. Artichokes are also a good source of digestive fibre.

Beetroot is a good source of digestive supportive fibre, which is great if your child has constipation. It has the added benefits of free-radical scavenging vitamin C and copper, bone-healthy magnesium and energy-producing iron and phosphorus. It has antioxidant properties and anti-inflammatory benefits and good amounts of folate, and is an excellent source of the antioxidant manganese and of potassium.

Beetroot soup

1 onion
2 garlic cloves
2 carrots
220g (8oz) beetroot
220g (8oz) potato
220g (8oz) cabbage
1 tablespoon olive oil

Peel and chop or slice all the vegetables. Fry the onion and the garlic in the oil and then add all the other vegetables. Stir and allow to cook gently for 10 minutes, then pour in a pint (500ml/2 cups) of water, bring to the boil and simmer for 30 minutes. Liquidize in a blender to make a smooth soup.

Carrot & Nutmeg Sauce

25g (1oz) butter
1 onion, peeled & chopped
750g (1½lb) carrots, scrubbed & chopped
pinch sea salt
1 teaspoon honey
1 teaspoon nutmeg
150ml (⅔ cup) water

Gently sweat the onion in the butter. Add water and carrots and cook until they are soft (about 10 minutes). Whizz in a blender with the honey, nutmeg and salt. If you add more water, it can also be a soup.

Used in small dosages, nutmeg can reduce flatulence, aid digestion, improve the appetite and treat diarrhoea, vomiting and nausea.

This sauce is nice poured over vegetables and potatoes, or as a small puree on its own if appetite isn't great. To make a more substantial dish, add a savoury crumble topping.

Savoury Crumble

Oats are calming and provide good fibre, which will help with constipation.

110g (1¼ cups) jumbo oats
55g (2oz) flaked almonds
½ teaspoon thyme
1 tablespoon olive oil

Put oats and oil in bowl together and mix until the oats are coated in oil, then add in the almonds and thyme. Put on top of the moist vegetable mixture, (the oats will absorb some of the juices) and bake at 200C (400F/Gas 6) for 20 minutes, until crisp and brown.

Stetson Baked Beans

2 tablespoons olive oil
1 onion, peeled & sliced
2 garlic cloves, crushed
½ teaspoon thyme
2 tablespoons tomato puree
200g (8oz) chopped tomatoes
2 teaspoons caster sugar
400g/1 tin red kidney beans in water
200ml (¾ cup) vegetable stock

Gently cook the onion, garlic and thyme in oil until soft. Drain and rinse the beans, then add with all the other ingredients to the pan, bring to the boil and simmer for 30 minutes stirring occasionally. If it gets too dry add more water.

Stetson Sauce

3 tablespoons olive oil
1 onion, peeled & sliced
2 garlic cloves, crushed
1 red pepper, finely chopped
400g /1 tin red kidney beans in water 2 tomatoes, chopped
little squirt of bbq or chilli sauce

Gently cook the vegetables in the oil. Drain and rinse the beans, then add the beans and bbq sauce to the vegetables; simmer for 10 minutes, until pulpy. Serve with rice.

All beans and legumes, lentils and wholegrains provide good amounts of dietary fibre, essential to ease constipation, so give your little cowboys and cowgirls some, ranch style.

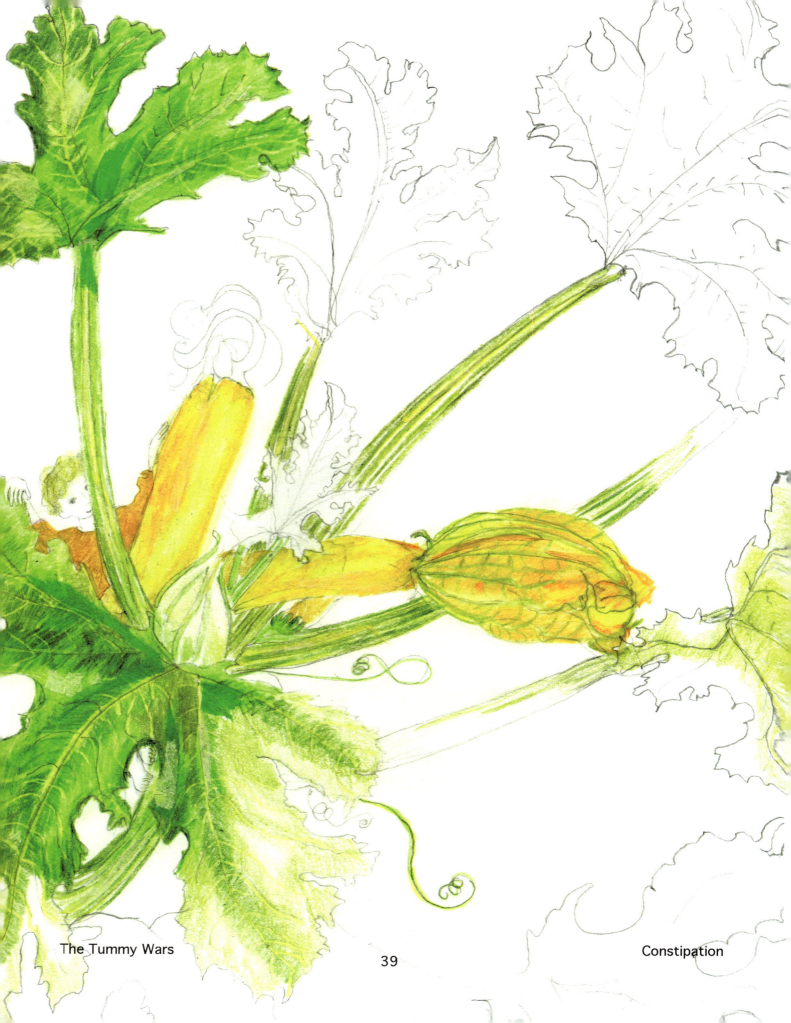

Courgette & Almond Stuffing

2 large courgettes/ zucchini
1 tablespoon olive oil
1 onion, sliced
2 garlic cloves, crushed
250g (2½ cups) ground almonds
1 tomato, chopped

Preheat oven to 200C (400F/Gas 6).

Halve courgettes lengthwise and scoop out the fleshy inside (put aside for the stuffing), then parboil them for a couple of minutes. Remove from pan and blot dry with kitchen towel.

For the stuffing, fry the onion, garlic, tomato and courgette flesh until glistening and golden, then add the almonds, mix together, remove from heat and stuff mixture into the courgette scoops. Cook in the oven for 20 minutes.

Leek with Potatoes, Garlic & Thyme

2 tablespoons olive oil
1 onion, sliced
2 garlic cloves, crushed
3 large potatoes, peeled & chopped
2 leeks, washed & sliced
½ teaspoon thyme
200ml (¾ cup) stock or bouillon

Heat the oil in a heavy based saucepan and sweat the onion. Add the other ingredients and water or stock, stir, cover and simmer with lid on for 20 minutes, until all vegetables are very tender.

Figs, Prunes, Pears & Apple

Chop 4 figs, 4 prunes, 1 large apple and 1 pear.

Put into a saucepan with 250ml (1 cup) weak camomile tea or water, a stick of cinnamon and a clove. Bring to the boil, then simmer on a low heat until the fruits are all soft and glossy. Remove the clove and cinnamon stick. Can be served hot, warm or cold, with probiotic (live) plain Greek-style yogurt. Add manuka honey if you wish.

Figs and prunes have been used to ease constipation for years They have lots of dietary fibre and a sweet taste. You could use prune juice as a drink or to sweeten porridge.

Pear & Ginger Crumble

4 pears, peeled, decored & sliced
1 teaspoon grated root ginger
75g (⅓ cup) butter
100g (½ cup) dark muscovado sugar
handful of jumbo oats
1 tablespoon sesame seeds
1 tablespoon wheatgerm
100g (4oz) quinoa flour or flakes

Preheat oven to 190C (375F/Gas 5). Combine the pear and ginger together and put in a shallow ovenproof dish. Mix the other ingredients into a crumble and sprinkle over the pear. Bake for 30 minutes until the crumble is brown.

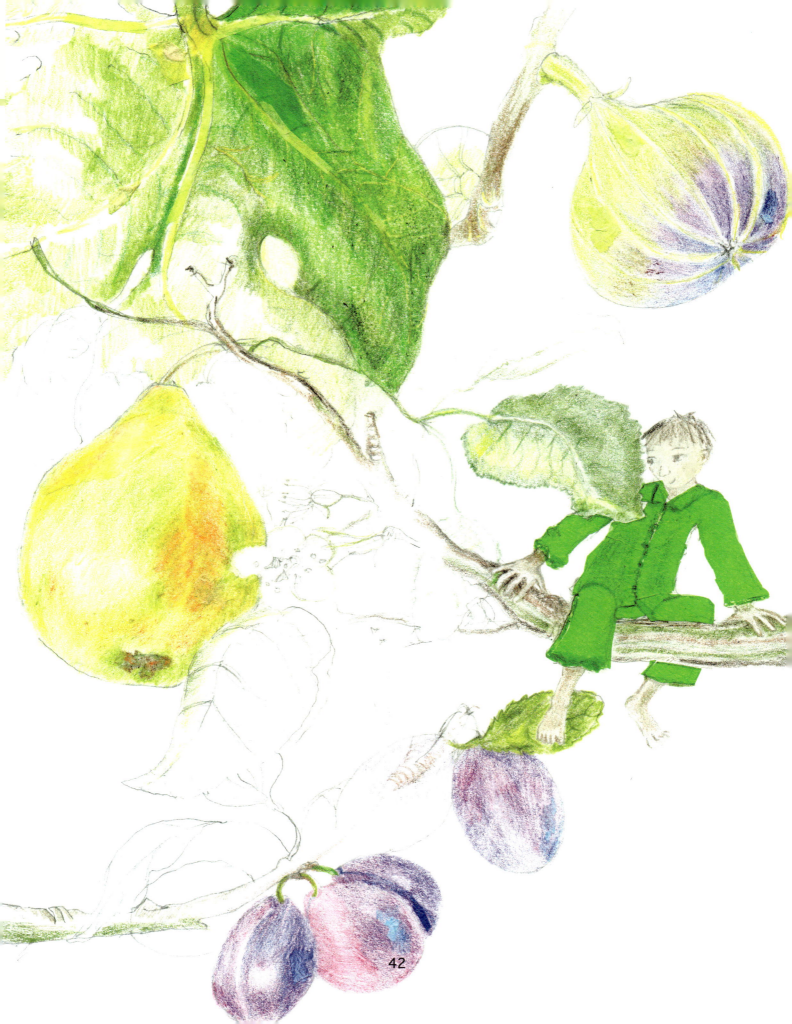

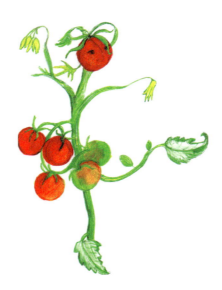

LYCOPENE is a carotenoid; it gives colour to carrots, squash, tomatoes, sweet potatoes, watermelon, papaya, pink grapefruit, pink guava, red peppers, rosehip & wolfberry/goji berry. It is a powerful antioxidant & protects against disease. It is the most powerful of the carotenoids to disarm the free radicals.

BETA CAROTENE is a form of vitamin A. It is a bright orange colour & is found in sweet potatoes, mangoes, papaya, carrots, squashes & green leafy vegetables like spinach & kale. Beta carotene increases the activity of the body's natural killer cells, is great for fighting off infections & is an anti-inflammatory antioxidant.

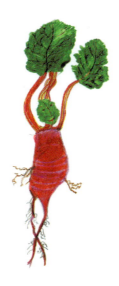

Return of the Tummy Wars

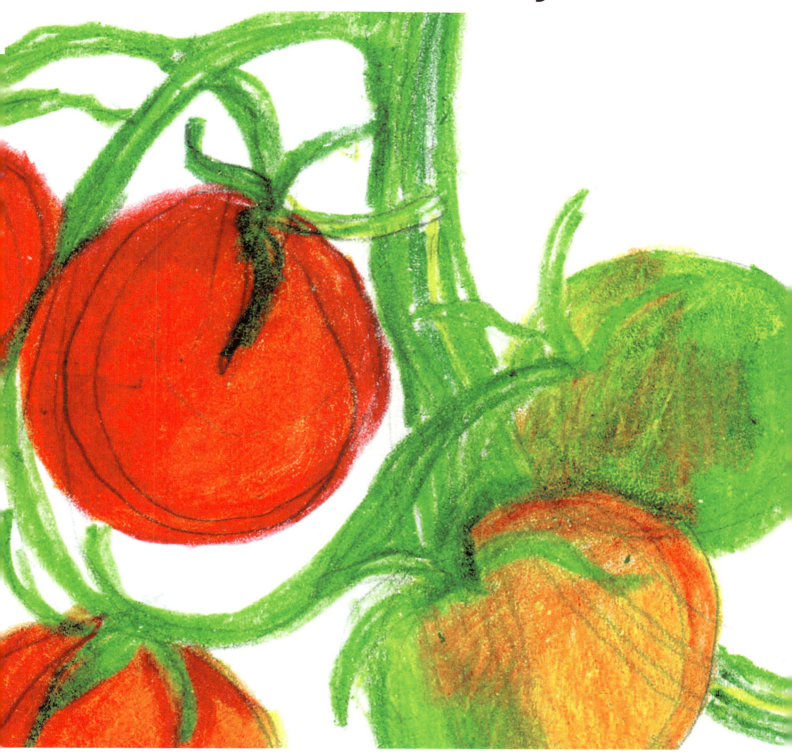

Recipes to Help with Diarrhoea & Vomiting

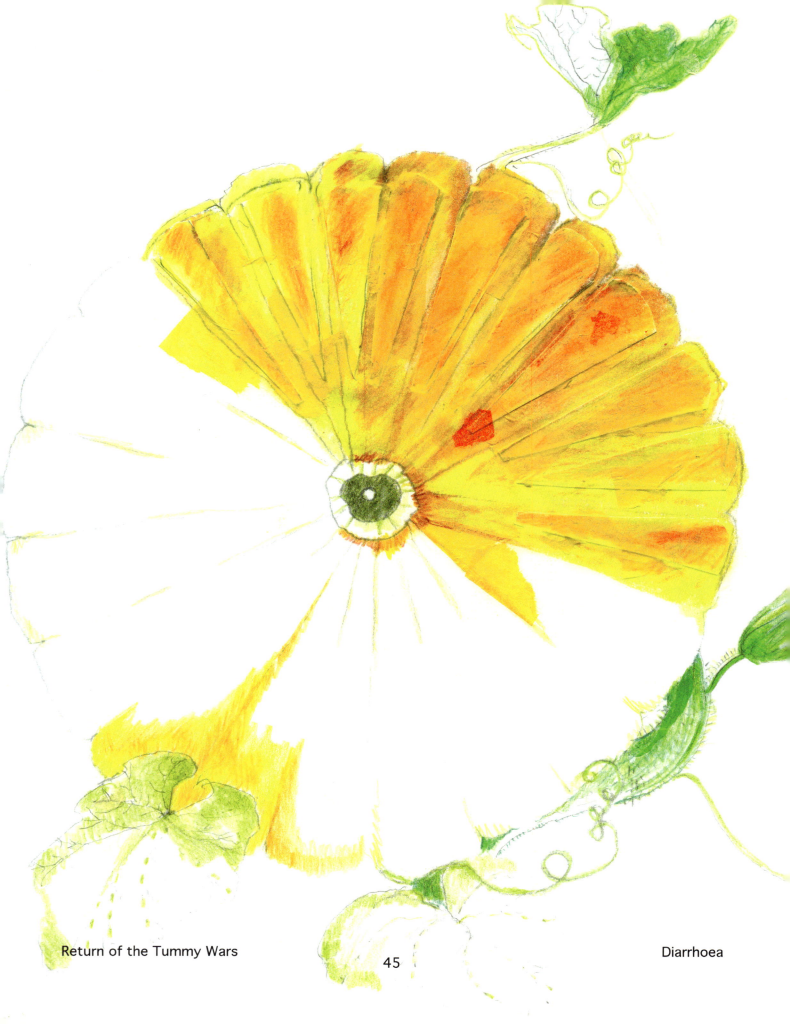

Recipes To Help with Diarrhoea

Simplest Soup

220g (8oz) each pumpkin, carrots, courgettes, peeled & chopped
1 litre (4 cups) water
handful of fresh sage
2 tablespoons olive oil

Sweat pumpkin and carrots in olive oil for about 10 minutes. Cover with a litre of water and simmer for a further 10 minutes. Add courgettes and sage, cook for another 5 minutes and whizz in a blender until smooth.

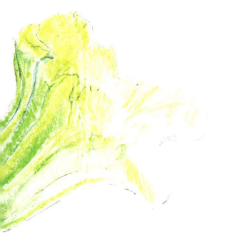

Pumpkin & Tofu Puree

500g (1lb) pumpkin, peeled & de-seeded
250g (9oz) firm tofu, drained

Steam, boil or roast the pumpkin pieces until cooked, then put in the blender with the tofu. Whizz until smooth and creamy (it may curdle at first). Add cardamom and apple juice for a sweet version, or garlic and nutmeg for a savoury puree.

Foods that are good for you if you have diarrhoea are brown rice, millet, pumpkin, carrot, apple, courgette and tofu. Camomile, aniseed, rosehip, hibiscus and lemon verbena teas are also helpful. Essential oils of geranium, camomile, sandalwood, frankincense and lavender can be massaged into the abdomen with a clockwise motion.

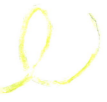

Baked Apple

1 eating apple, cored
1 tablespoon blackberries
1 small teaspoon molasses
pinch ground cinnamon & cloves

Preheat oven to 190C (375F/Gas 5).

Put the apple in an oven-proof dish.
Mix the other ingredients together in a
separate bowl. Fill the cored-out apple
with the blackberries, squish them in. Put
enough water in the bottom of the dish so
that the apple doesn't dry out, and bake
for 35 minutes until the apple is very soft.

Stewed Apple with Cloves & Molasses

1 bag eating apples, peeled & cored
225ml (1 cup) weak camomile tea/ water
1 level teaspoon molasses
1 clove

Put apples and camomile tea or water in
saucepan and bring to the boil. Add the
clove, simmer until soft, remove the clove
and stir in the molasses.

Stewed apple is good for diarrhoea, and
molasses has iron which helps produce
white blood cells and antibodies to fight off
infections. Camomile soothes the stomach.

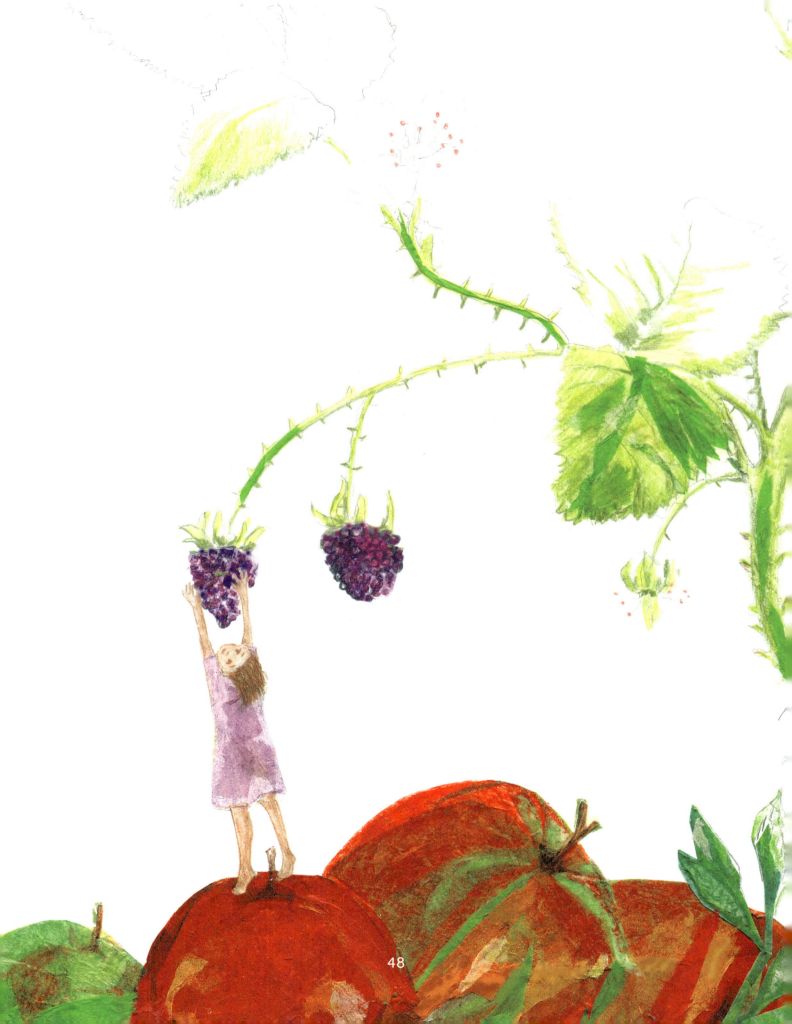

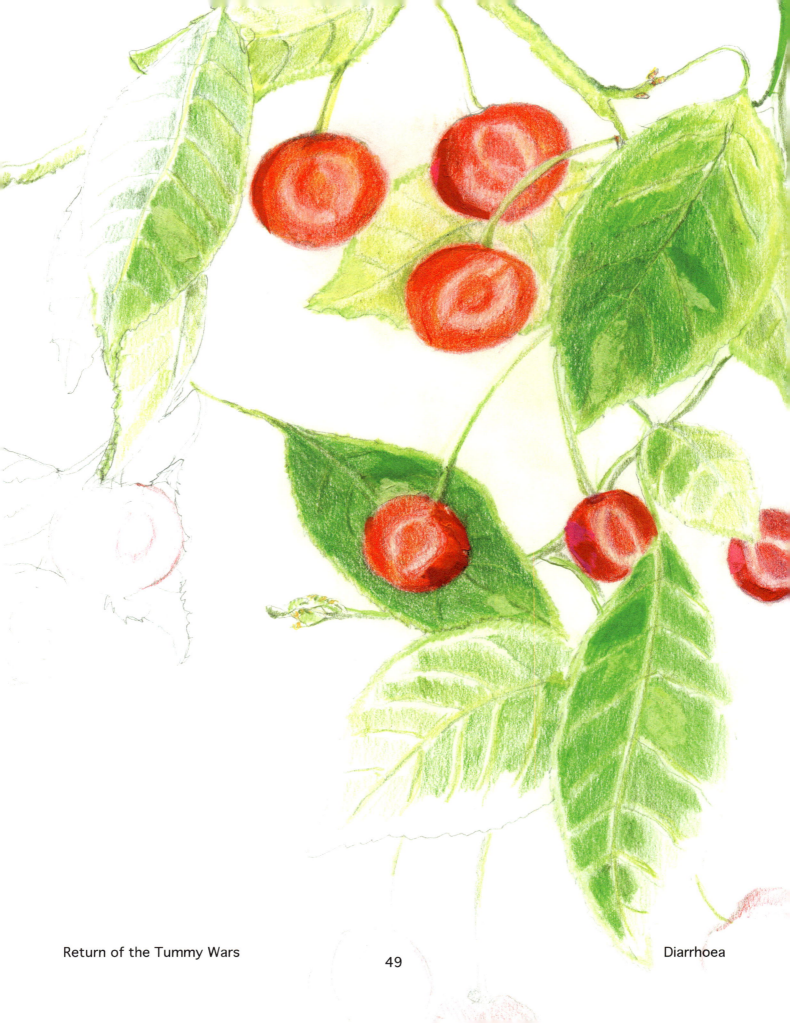

49

Rehydrate

Often after a bout of diarrhoea your child will need some gentle rehydration.
Coconut water is a very good rehydrator; it has lots of naturally occurring electrolytes and potassium. Watermelon is another good hydrator.

Watermelon & Ginger Ice

½ watermelon cut into chunks
2 tablespoons ginger cordial

Whizz up the watermelon in a blender until smooth. Mix in the cordial, put into a freezable shallow container and freeze for 3 hours. During the first hour, stir every 20 minutes to break up the particles.

Watermelon will rehydrate and ginger will help to settle the tum.

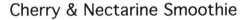

Cherry & Nectarine Smoothie

2 ripe frozen bananas, peeled
10 de-stoned cherries
2 nectarines, peeled & stoned
1 teaspoon of omega oil (or linseed/
hemp)

Whizz in a blender until smooth

Cherries are full of antioxidants to help infections, and nectarines have a high vitamin content. If you are fighting bacteria, these will help, as well as being hydrating.

Recipes To Help after Vomiting

Simple Rehydration Drink

1 litre (4 cups) water or weak herbal tea
600ml (2½ cups) pear or apple juice
1 teaspoon sea salt
1 tablespoon fructose or
½ tablespoon agave syrup

Mix everything together and drink.
Can be stored in the fridge for 2 days.

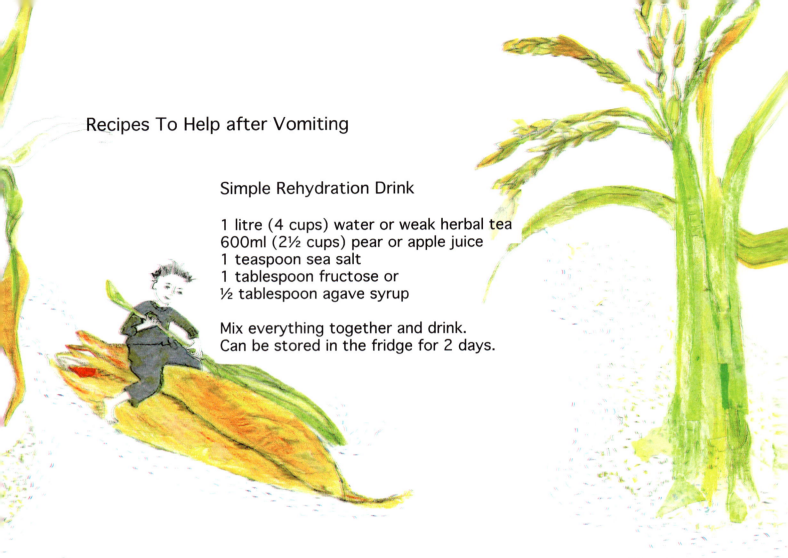

Rice Pudding

When your child feels up to eating something, a little of this gentle rice pudding might do the trick. Rice is easy to digest and the fruit will give a little energy.

80g (½ cup) basmati rice
1 tablespoon sultanas
1 tablespoon chopped dried apricots, peaches or pineapple
375ml (1 ½ cups) milk or nut milk
2 tablespoons maple syrup
1 teaspoon vanilla extract
1 large pinch cardamom, ginger & cinnamon

One teaspoon of cinnamon contains as many antioxidants as a cup of pomegranate juice or half a cup of blueberries.

Preheat oven to 180C (350F/Gas 4). Grease a 15x15cm or 6x6inch deep baking dish with a little butter. Sprinkle the rice and dried fruit into the dish. Whisk all the other ingredients in a bowl and pour over the rice. Bake for 45 minutes until it becomes firm. Serve warm, perhaps with some fruit compote or bio greek yogurt.

Banana & Currant Cake

4 ripe bananas, mashed
2 eggs, beaten
1 teaspoon mixed spice
75g (½ cup) currants or other dried fruit
75g (⅓ cup) butter
220g (1¾ cups) self-raising flour

Preheat the oven to 180C (350F/ Gas 4). Mix the eggs and the bananas together in a bowl. Add the other ingredients and stir well. Put into a lined and oiled loaf tin, and bake for 40 minutes until cooked.

Bananas can help replace potassium. Puree, smoothie or cook, however preferred.

Banana Smoothie

1 frozen banana
75g (½ cup) frozen blueberries
220ml (1 cup) soya/quinoa/coconut or almond milk.

Whizz all together for a refreshing drink.

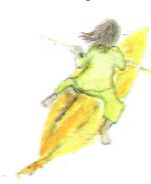

Banana Ice-Cream

2 ripe bananas
75g (¾ cup) ground cashew nuts
1 tablespoon maple or agave syrup
1 teaspoon lecithin granules
225ml (1 cup) nut milk

Blend everything together and freeze in a shallow container. Mix with a fork after an hour of freezing. Take out of freezer 5 minutes before serving.

Banana Nut Snack

Squish a ripe banana and put on top of an oat biscuit, which is topped with a nut butter (almond, hazelnut, walnut, pecan), for a nutrient-dense snack.

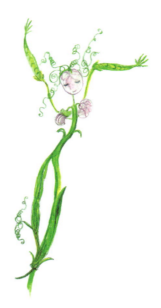

ZEAXANTHIN is a carotenoid, found in yellow corn, kiwi fruit, paprika, red peppers & saffron. It is also in eggs, turnips, goji berries, kale, green leafy vegetables, lettuce, broccoli, courgettes, peas & sprouts. It is similar to lutein & is a powerful antioxidant which protects the body from the damage caused by free radicals.

LUTEIN is a carotenoid, it comes from the Latin word meaning yellow so not surprisingly is found in carrots, squash & orange & yellow fruits such as apricots, mango & peach. It is also found in egg yolk & green leafy vegetables like spinach, kale, sprouts, broccoli, peas & courgettes. It is an efficient scavenger of free radicals & also protects the eyes.

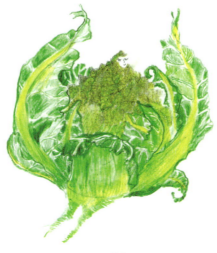

Healthy Tums

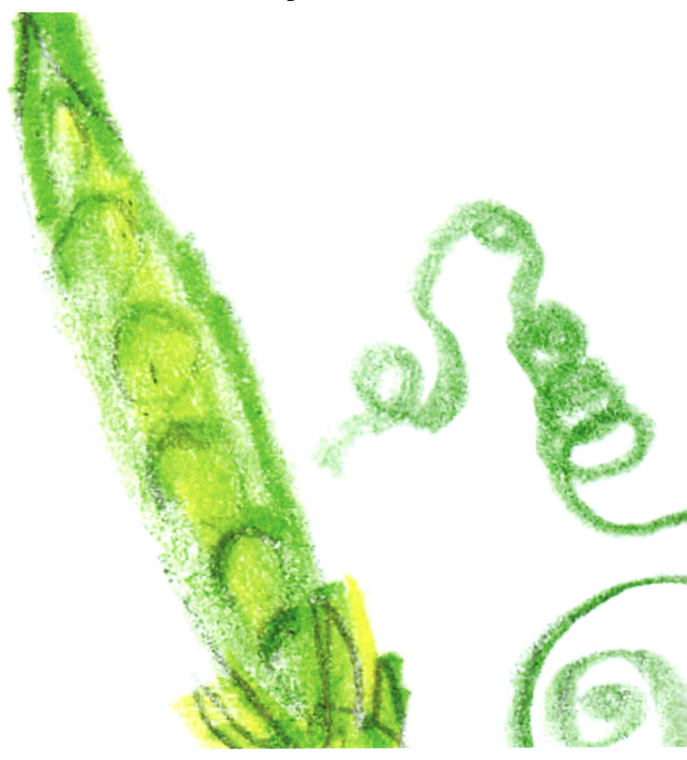

Recipes to Build Good Gut Bacteria

Recipes to Repair Gut Bacteria

These recipes will help repair the gut flora after an illness or after taking medication. The gut flora is an important part of the immune system, and plays lots of roles in keeping us healthy and nourished. These bacteria are the "live", "probiotic" bacteria that are found in yogurts. When we are ill, stressed or take medication, these bacteria can be damaged, depleted or wiped out.

To start the road to recovery, it is important to replenish the environment of the gut. There are two ways of doing this. One is to take in the bacteria, either with fermented foods such as yogurt, cottage cheese, miso, shoyu, sauerkraut, sourdough bread, especially those cultured with Lactobacillus or bifidobacteria or supplementation (Lactobacillus and Bifidobacteria acidophilus).

The second way is to provide the food that these bacteria live off. They live off sugars called fructo-oligo-saccharides, or FOS for short, which is sometimes known as a prebiotic. FOS are found in bananas, cabbage, barley, fruit, garlic, onions, soybeans, wheat and jerusalem artichokes, (see recipe for jerusalem artichoke soup in Chapter 2).

Avocado & Cottage Cheese Smoothie

220g (8oz) cottage cheese
440ml (1¾ cup) soya or rice milk
½ ripe avocado, diced
1 tablespoon organic agave nectar
4 ice cubes (½ cup) crushed ice

Blend the cottage cheese and ½ cup of soya milk in a blender until smooth. Add the avocado. Cover and blend until fairly smooth, about 30 seconds. Add the remaining soya milk and the agave nectar, cover and blend for 10 seconds. Add the ice; cover and blend until the smoothie is thick and the ice has melted.

Delicious avocados are full of anti-inflammatory omega 9 fat, high in antioxidants (carotenoid, lutein, zeaxanthin, alpha-carotene and beta-carotene) and vitamin E which is an antioxidant and helps repair the gut wall.

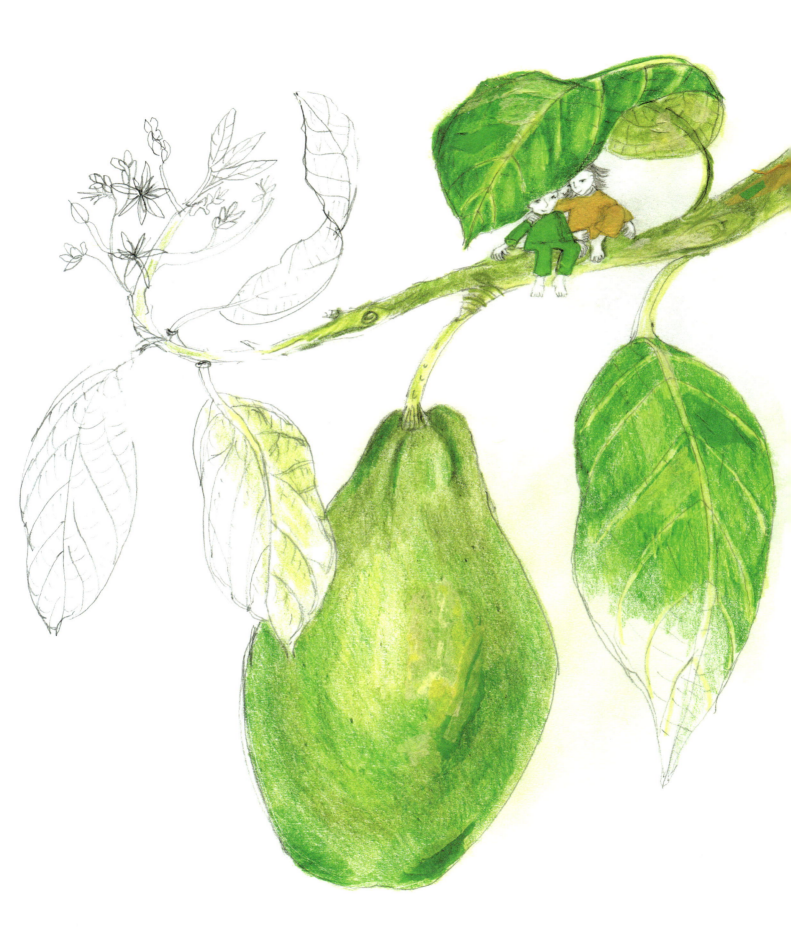

Cabbage Wraps

12 large green cabbage leaves
200g (7oz) firm plain tofu, finely sliced
230g (8oz) minced lean pork
150g (5oz)spring onions, finely sliced
1 large carrot, grated
50g (2oz) shiitake mushrooms, finely sliced
1 teaspoon sesame oil
2 tablespoons rice vinegar or mirin
½ teaspoon salt
½ teaspoon sugar
500ml (2 cups) vegetable stock
1 tablespoon light soy sauce

Blanche the cabbage leaves by bringing a large pan of boiling water to the boil and dipping them in for about 10 seconds; this makes them pliable. Drain and set aside.

Place the pork, tofu, spring onions, carrot and mushrooms in a bowl. Mix with the sesame oil, mirin, salt or sugar. Put some of the pork mixture in the middle of a flat cabbage leaf. Fold the stem end over, tuck in the sides and roll up. Secure with a tooth pick. Place the cabbage rolls in a saucepan, cover with the stock and soy sauce, then heat until nearly boiling. Simmer moderately for 15 minutes, turning once. Remove the cabbage rolls from the stock and serve.

Cabbage and Tofu help to feed the good gut bacteria. Shiitake mushrooms contain the powerful antioxidant L-ergothioneine and lentinan. Among lentinan's healing benefits is its ability to power up the immune system, which strengthens its ability to fight infection and disease.

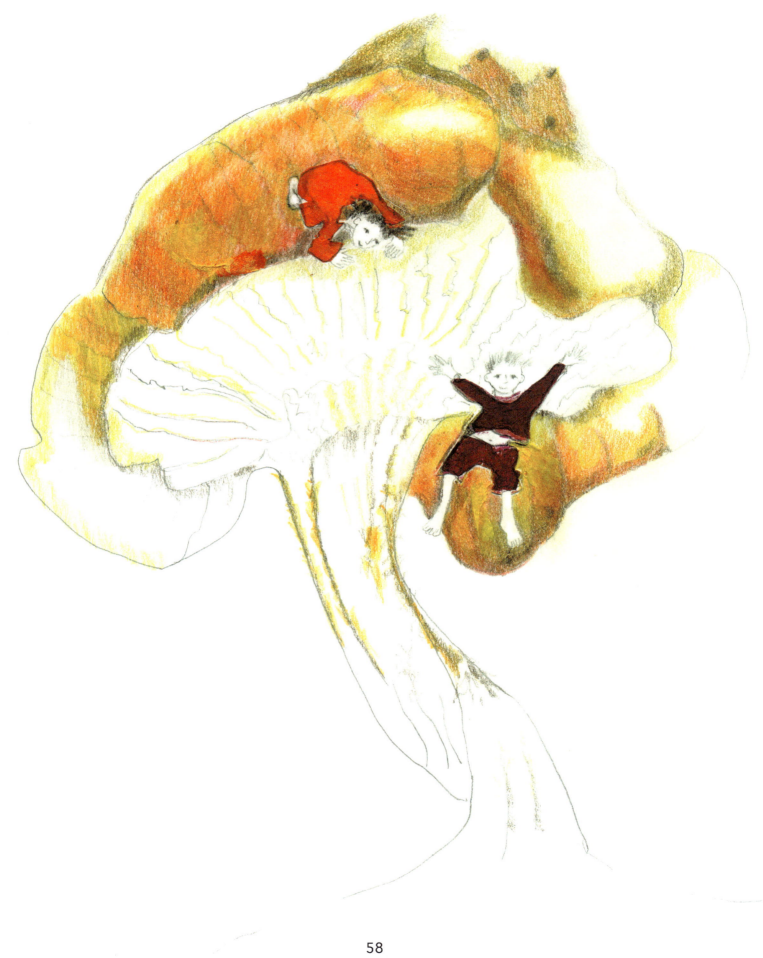

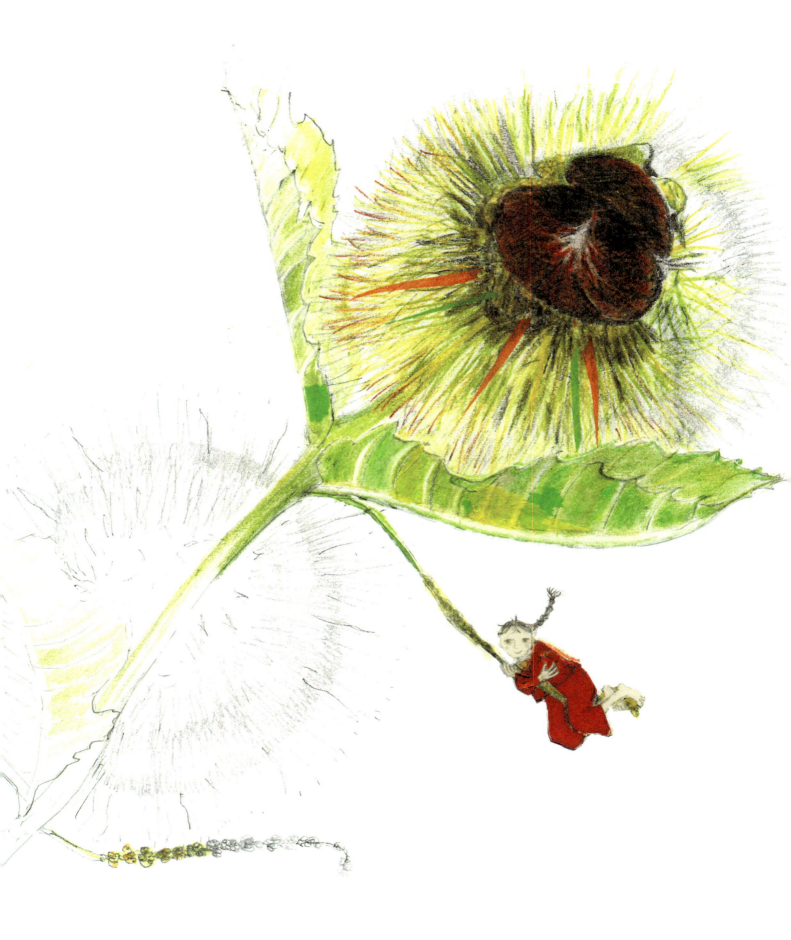

Barley & Chestnut Pudding

1 tin whole chestnuts
2 eggs
7 tablespoons barley flour
2 tablespoons agave syrup
¾ teaspoon baking powder
handful golden raisins or pitted prunes cut into small pieces

Puree the tin of chestnuts with its liquid in a blender. When smooth, transfer to a bowl and add the other ingredients; pour into an oiled cake tin and bake for 25 minutes at 200C (400F/Gas 6).

Barley is nutrient-dense and a great provider of the food for good gut bacteria.

Chestnuts are low in fat and high in dietary fibre; they are a powerhouse of nutrients with large amounts of manganese, potassium, copper, phosphorus, magnesium and iron. Zinc and calcium are also present in small amounts. They have high amounts of vitamin C, (a powerful antioxidant), and the B vitamins which provide energy.

Probiotic yogurt has lots of good bacteria to help the gut, and maple syrup is a good source of manganese and zinc, both of which are important for the healthy function of the immune system. Manganese can help lessen inflammation because it is part of the wonderful antioxidant, superoxide dismutase (or SOD for short).

Chestnut & Almond Pudding

175g (1⅓ cups) chestnut flour
1 litre (4 cups) almond milk
3 to 5 tablespoons honey
(or agave nectar or maple syrup)
1 pot probiotic Greek-style yogurt

Pour almond milk in a saucepan and lightly sift in flour a little at a time to keep smooth, constantly mixing with a wooden spoon. Keep over a low heat, stir until thickened. When thick, gradually add the honey and simmer for 5 minutes, stirring all the time. Pour into dessert dish and chill before serving with a dollop of yogurt.

Banana & Cinnamon Pudding

350g (12oz) rice flakes
280ml (1⅛ cup) rice milk
2 ripe bananas, mashed up with a fork
handful of raisins

Soak the rice flakes in a bowl with the rice milk, add the other ingredients and then pour into an oiled cake tin.

Bake at 200C (400F/Gas 6) for 30 minutes.

Cinnamon Cover

1 ½ tablespoons of rice cream (farina)
1 ½ teaspoons ground cinnamon
375ml (1½ cups) soya milk
2 tablespoons agave syrup
vanilla pod, seeds removed

Slowly heat the farina, vanilla and cinnamon in a saucepan. Add the soya milk, stir until thickened, (the consistency should be that the back of a spoon is coated, while remaining fluid). Remove from heat, add syrup and cool. Cover the banana cake with the cinnamon sauce to serve.

A bunch of bananas is called a "hand".

Each banana is a good source of vitamin B6, vitamin C, manganese, potassium and dietary fibre. B6 is essential to help you digest proteins and use them for growth and repair, and is a natural anti-depressant! Manganese helps antioxidants work and reduces cell damage, and potassium can help your gut work properly.

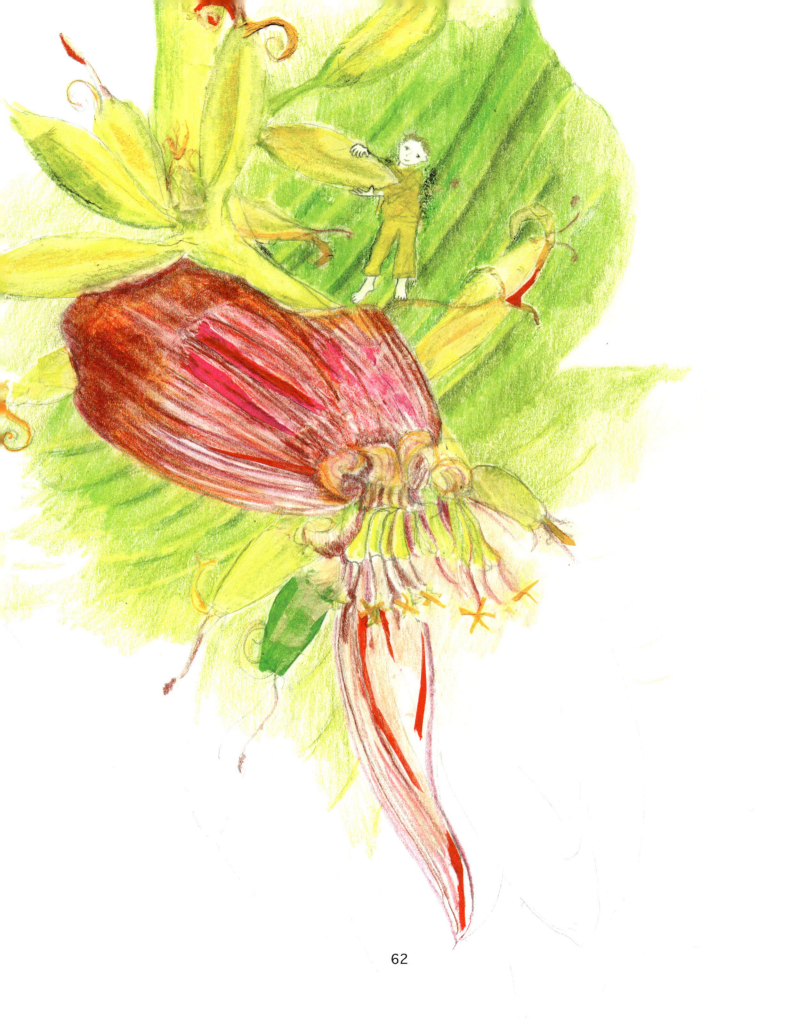

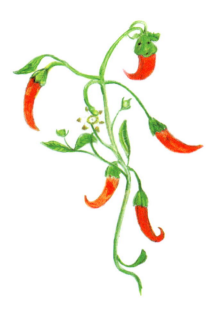

PIPERINE & CAPSICUM. Piperine is an alkaloid & it makes the hotness of the pepper; capsicum is the active component of chilli peppers. They help curcumin work & can help lessen pain, heat the body up & reduce inflammation in ear inflections.

GENISTEIN is an isoflavone. It is found in fava or broad beans, endamame or soy beans & soya products such as milk or tofu, kudzu & coffee. It is an antioxidant, helps the body to detoxify & is anthelmintic, (it kills parasitic worms).

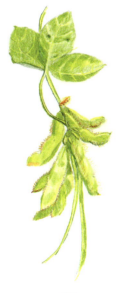

Get Better Baths & Soothing Soaks

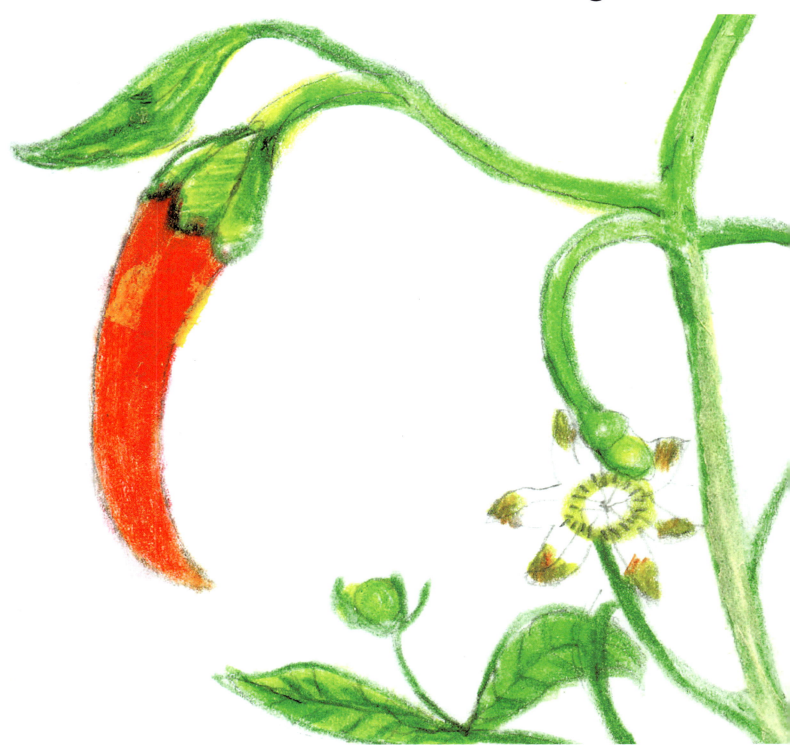

Warming Baths for Colds, Relaxing Baths to Ease Tension & Soothing Baths for Stomach Aches

Get Better Baths & Soothing Soaks

Sprinkle a few sprigs of the following herbs or spices into a nicely hot bath, let them steep for at least 5 or 10 minutes and either remove them from the bath or leave in for your child to explore.
Remove sprigs before pulling the plug to avoid blocking the drains.

If the thought of bits of plants in the bath seems too messy then put them in a pop sock or old tights to make a "muslin" pouch.

Lavender flowers are antiseptic, antibacterial and healing. They are also soothing and help induce calm sleep. However too many can be stimulating rather than sedative.

A sprig of rosemary - rejuvenating and warming.

Rosehip and hibiscus tea bags or loose tea. Lovely colour, soothing and beautiful.

Bay leaves help get rid of mucus and soothe aching limbs.

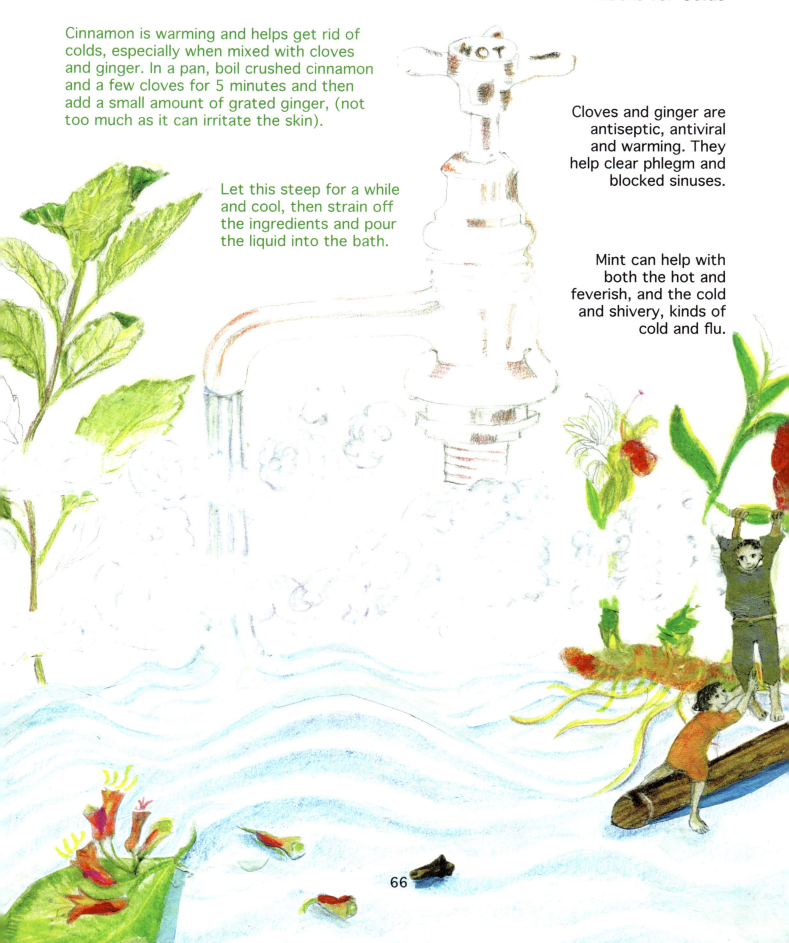

Cinnamon is warming and helps get rid of colds, especially when mixed with cloves and ginger. In a pan, boil crushed cinnamon and a few cloves for 5 minutes and then add a small amount of grated ginger, (not too much as it can irritate the skin).

Cloves and ginger are antiseptic, antiviral and warming. They help clear phlegm and blocked sinuses.

Let this steep for a while and cool, then strain off the ingredients and pour the liquid into the bath.

Mint can help with both the hot and feverish, and the cold and shivery, kinds of cold and flu.

66

Baths for Colds

Basil is antibacterial and antiparasitic; it helps to expel a head cold or fever.

Oregano and Marjoram can help ease the "shivery" type of cold; with natural antibiotic and spasmodic action, they help to relieve coughs.

Thyme and Lemon Thyme are useful in calming heat and feverishness, help to expel mucus and clear blocked sinuses.

Sage strengthens lungs and has properties that support the immune system.

Soothing Recipe for Stomach Aches

Boil in a saucepan cardamom seeds, (split open the pods to release the seeds), some coriander, cumin and slightly crushed fennel seeds. Boil for 5 minutes and leave to steep and cool. Strain off seeds and pour liquid into the bath. All these spices can help calm stomach cramps and upsets.

Camomile helps with stomach upsets - you can use a couple of teabags if you don't have fresh camomile.

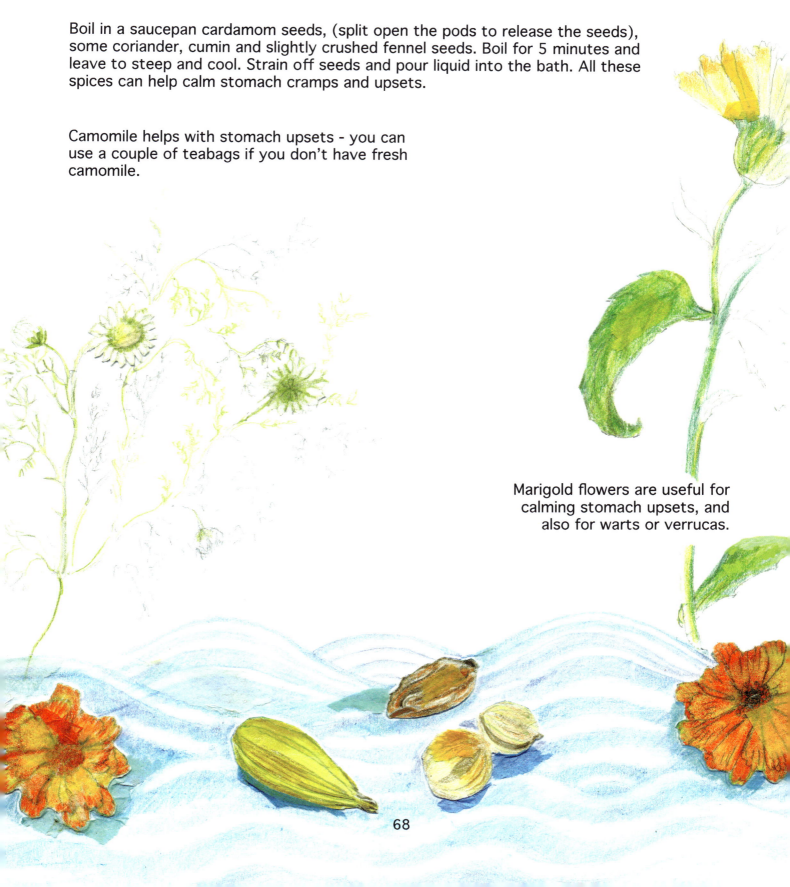

Marigold flowers are useful for calming stomach upsets, and also for warts or verrucas.

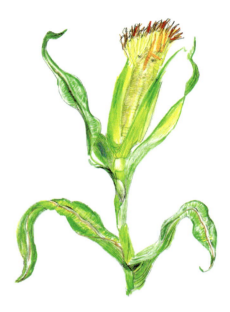

CURCUMIN is a polyphenol, found in members of the ginger family: ginger, turmeric, mustard, corn & yellow peppers. It is a free radical scavenger & antioxidant, antiviral & antifungal. It likes to work with piperine & capsicum - found in peppers, they help to make the yellow coloured curcumin work.

MYRICETIN is a flavonol found in grapes, berries, herbs, fruit & vegetables. The best source is walnuts. It is a protective antioxidant thought to lower LDL cholesterol & protect against certain cancers.

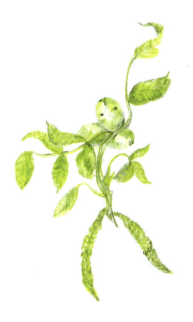

Broken Arms & Other Nasty Shocks

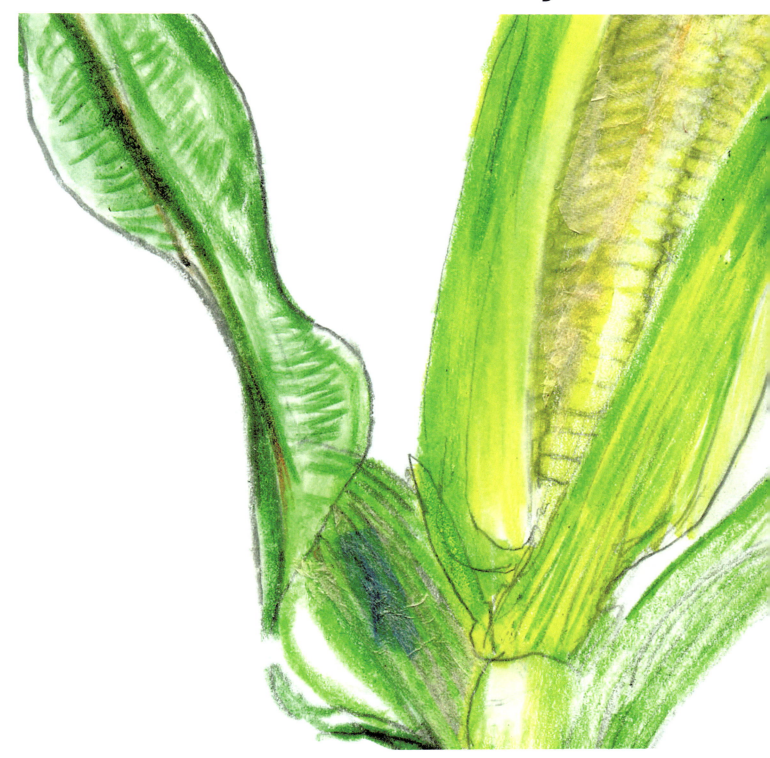

Recipes to Help Heal

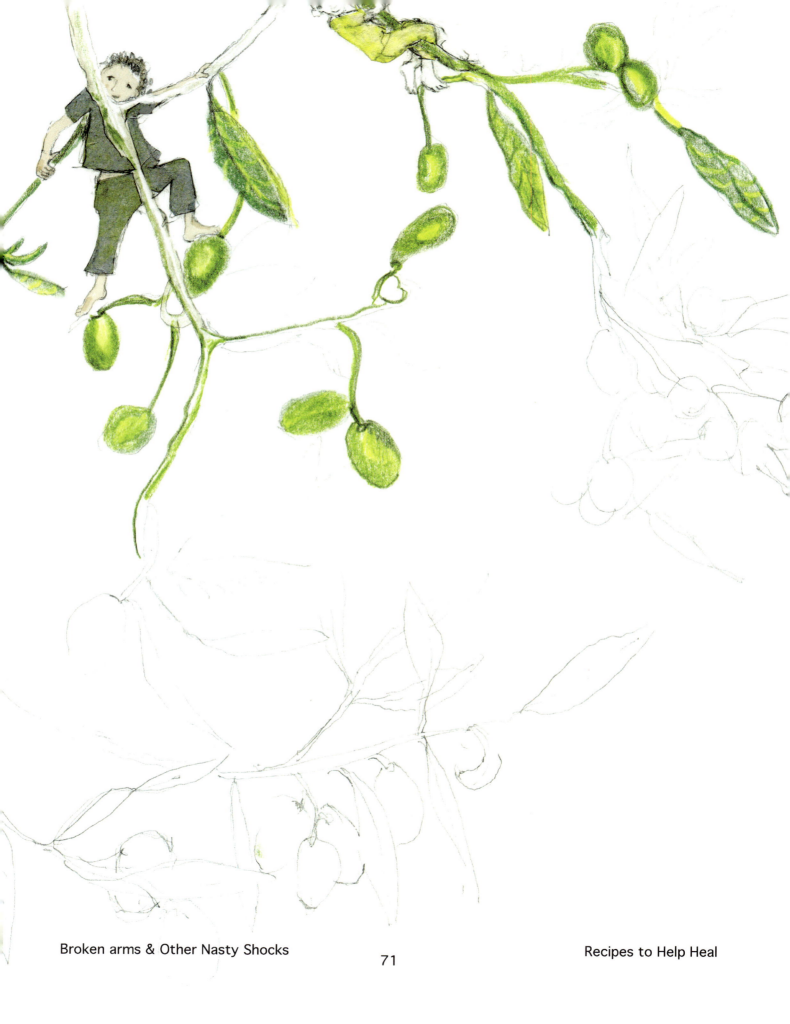

How to Heal

Broken bones, sprains, bruising, cuts and grazes all need nutrients that help them heal and which are anti-inflammatory. In this chapter, you will find recipes that combine several of these elements to help the body recover from surgery or an accident. The important nutrients for helping to heal are: protein, which encourages the body to rebuild; omega fats (essential fats from nuts, seeds and fish) to reduce inflammation; vitamin E which protects the omega fats; calcium, magnesium, phosphorus and vitamins D and K which are important for bone health; vitamin C which is essential for the formation and maintenance of connective tissue and wound healing; zinc which is needed when new tissue is formed (for example, when recovering from surgery or burns or when a wound is healing) and B vitamins which are useful for managing shock and stress.

Where does calcium come from if it doesn't come from a cow? Milk can be inflammatory and mucus-forming, so should be used sparingly with ill children. How does a cow make calcium? It only eats grass! Just as a cow makes calcium from grass, we humans can get calcium from green leafy vegetables, like broccoli, kale, watercress, spinach and okra. We also get calcium from fish, tofu and almonds. "Live" yogurt is another good source of calcium, and its active cultures produce some lactase enzyme which helps the absorption of nutrients.

Avocado Dip

1 ripe avocado, peeled and stoned
2 tablespoons cottage cheese or ½ pack of silken soy
squeeze of lemon
1 tablespoon olive oil

Whizz everything in a blender - dip with
carrot, cucumber, sweet pepper batons,
celery and tortilla chips.

For the tortilla chips, cut a tortilla into 8,
sprinkle with a little water and olive oil and
bake in oven for 5 minutes (until brittle) at
a high temperature.

A child-friendly take on guacamole, this has the added advantage of protein in the soy or cottage cheese. Avocado is full of beneficial fats (monounsaturated oleic acid which keeps skin soft and helps guard against damage), and vitamin E which will keep skin elastic and reduce scarring. The vegetables for the dip are full of antioxidants, vitamins and minerals.

Fish Pie with Sweet Mash

3 medium sweet potatoes
2 medium swedes
400ml (1⅔ cups) milk or soya milk
a knob of butter
1 medium leek, sliced
1 tablespoon olive oil
2 tablespoons ground oats
300g/3 fillets white fish or salmon (or both)
100g (4oz) shelled and de-veined prawns
a head of broccoli
large handful of peas or sweetcorn

Preheat oven to 180C (350F/Gas 4).

Peel and cut the sweet potato and swede into cubes, then steam for 10 minutes, until they can be smashed. Once cooked, drain and add butter and 100ml (⅓ cup) milk and mash well. Cook the leek with oil in an ovenproof pan for 4 minutes, and stir in the oats. Add 300ml (1⅓ cups) milk, stir until it thickens. Then add the fish, prawns and vegetables and cook together for about 5 minutes. Take off the heat and cover with the mash, transfer to the oven and bake for 25 minutes.

Oats contain a slow-releasing fibre which helps keep moods steady, helpful after a shock, and are a good source of energy, giving B vitamins, iron, zinc and vitamin E, which are useful for repair and growth. The fish provides proteins, vitamins, minerals and omega fats which will help the body to rebuild. Vitamin A from the sweet potatoes will help skin heal from cuts or grazes.

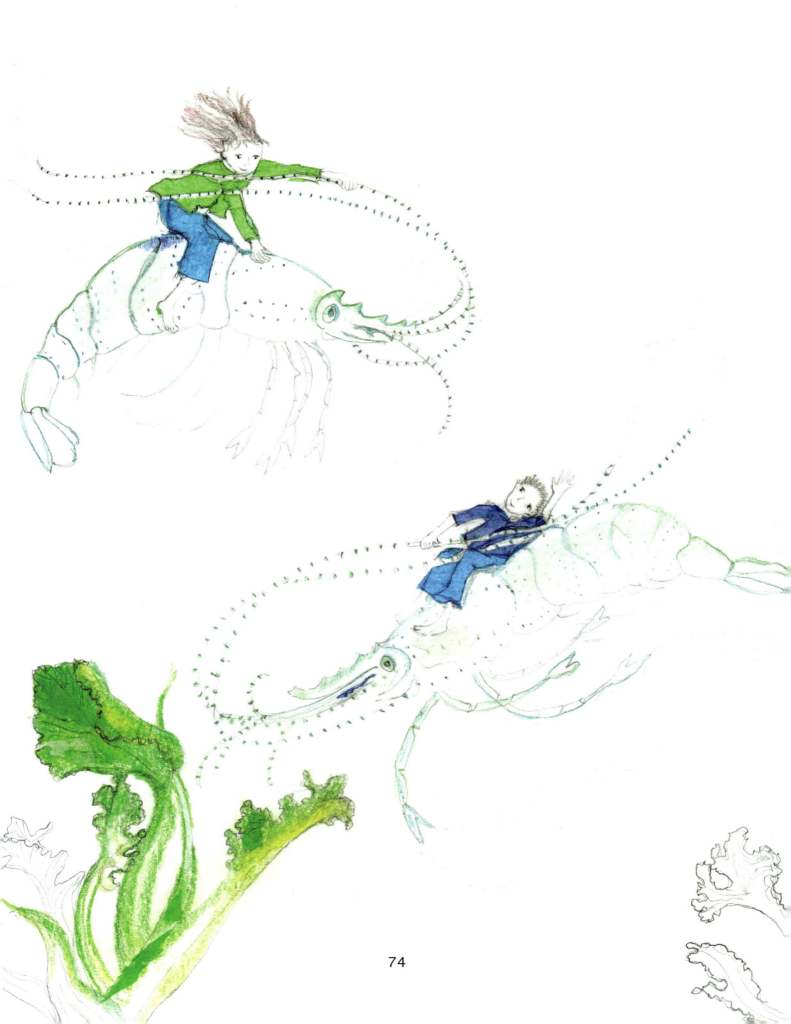

Beetroot & Fish Bliss

1 pack of precooked beetroot
3 cloves (1 teaspoon) garlic, crushed
2 teaspoons balsamic vinegar
4 thick salmon fillets, with skin
2 large potatoes, peeled and very finely sliced
500ml (2 cups) vegetable stock
2 tablespoons sunflower oil

Preheat oven to 200C.

Gently fry the potato in a frying pan until slightly browned, remove and place in the bottom of an oven proof dish, pour over the stock and place the fish fillets, skin side up, on top of the potatoes so the juices cook into the fish. Cover and cook for 20 minutes. In a blender whizz up the beetroot, garlic and vinegar, put into the oven to warm through. When the fish is cooked, remove cover from dish and place under the grill to crisp up the fish skin. Serve the potatoes with the fish on top and the beetroot around the side.

Sweet and enticing beetroot is a source of energy because of its high sugar content. It has gentle fibre which soothes the gut and protects the liver (important if medicines have been taken). Generally detoxifying and an immune support, it is brilliant food for recovery.

White fish will give protein for building, is easily digestible so supports the gut, and contains beneficial omega fats. Fish also contains B vitamins which help with growth and repair, energy levels and mood, and selenium and minerals with antioxidant properties, which can block the uptake of heavy metals such as mercury or lead.

Monkfish Splints for Broken Bones

For marinade:
2 tablespoons olive oil
1 tablespoon sesame oil
Juice of 1 lemon
Large handful chopped flat leaf parsley
1 large garlic clove, crushed

400g (1lb) monkfish fillets, cut in 3cm cubes
400g (1lb) preferred vegetables:
mushrooms, sweet peppers, sweet potatoes, baby corn, courgettes, aubergine, broccoli heads, cauliflower, small tomatoes

Mix marinade ingredients together, then marinade fish for at least 20 minutes. Cut all vegetables into the right size for skewers. Put all vegetables onto a baking tray, cover with a little marinade and grill slightly for several minutes to soften. When cool enough to handle, fold the aubergine and courgette pieces and thread all the vegetables onto the skewer, alternating with the monkfish. Grill kebabs for 5 minutes each side, turning regularly, until vegetables are blistered and fish cooked.

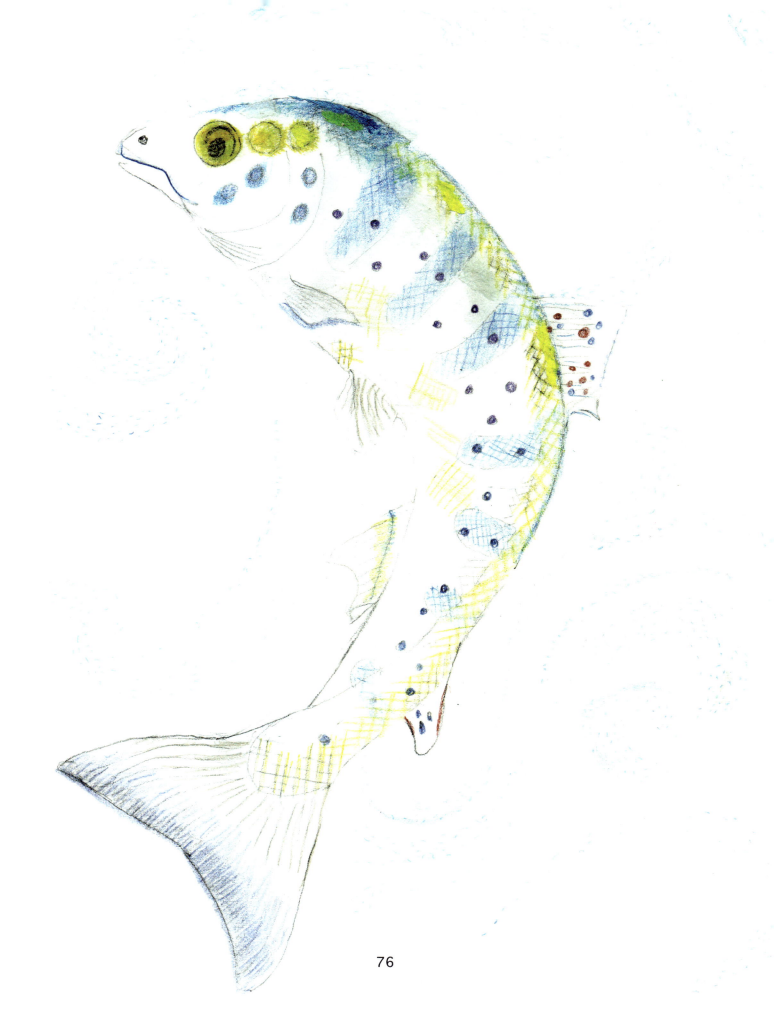

76

Pea Soup

1 onion, peeled & finely sliced
500g (2 cups) frozen or podded peas
750ml (3 cups) vegetable stock
2 tablespoons mint leaves, chopped
2 tablespoons parsley leaves, chopped

Heat a teaspoon of olive oil in a saucepan, add the onions and sweat until caramelized. Add the peas and the stock, boil and simmer for 10 minutes. Blend with the herb leaves until smooth. Serve warm, or chilled on a hot day.

Peas are a source of vitamin K, which is good for bone health, beta carotenes which support the immune system, B vitamins for growth, and protein and iron. Parsley is full of vitamins K, C and A, which all promote healthy growth and repair.

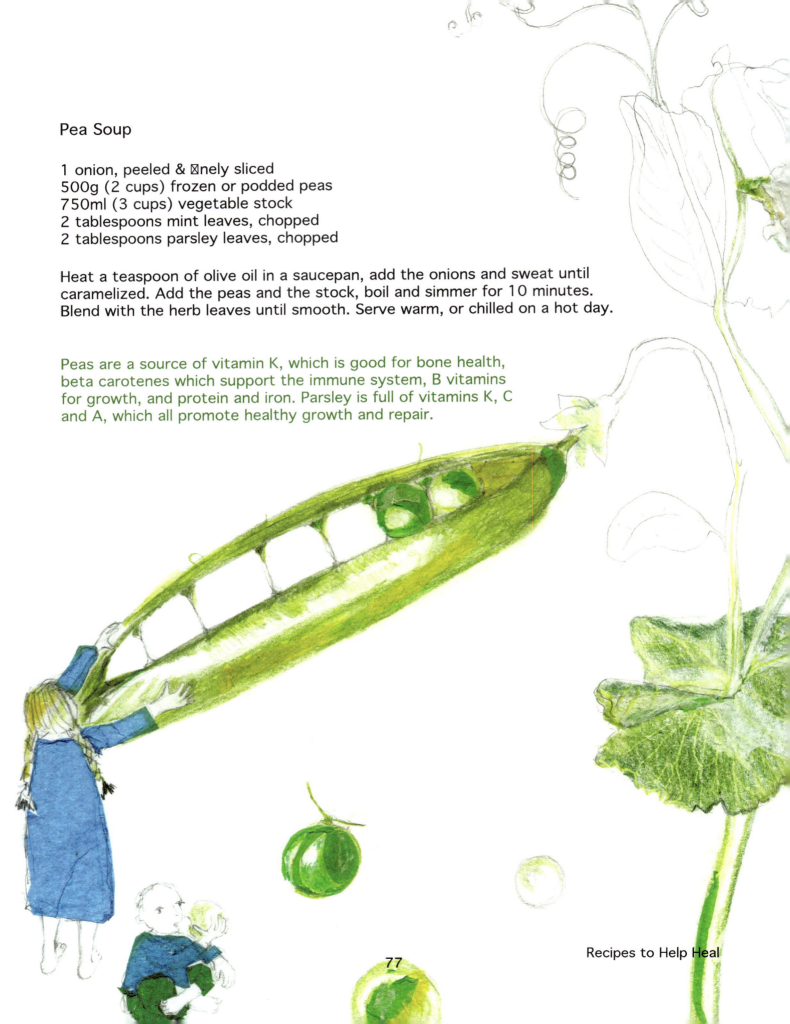

Recipes to Help Heal

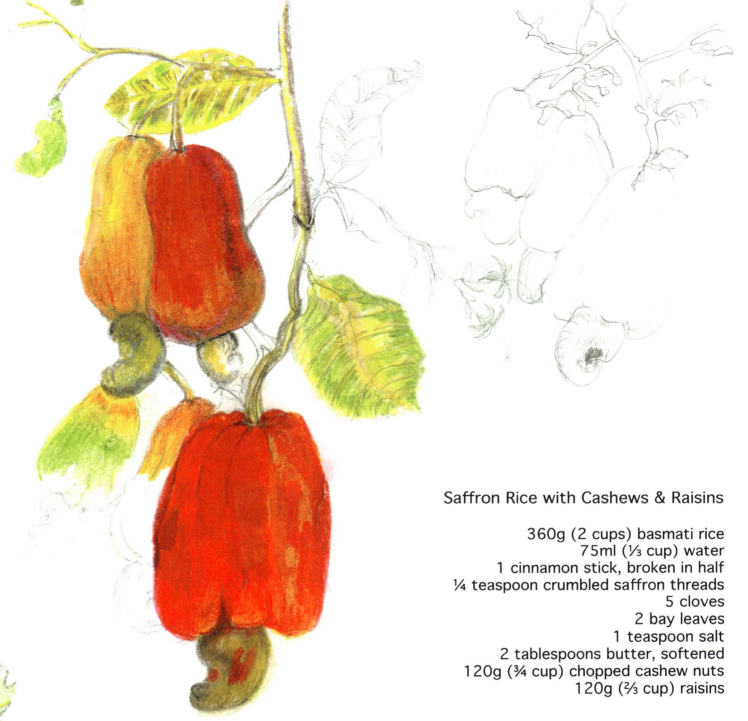

Saffron Rice with Cashews & Raisins

360g (2 cups) basmati rice
75ml (⅓ cup) water
1 cinnamon stick, broken in half
¼ teaspoon crumbled saffron threads
5 cloves
2 bay leaves
1 teaspoon salt
2 tablespoons butter, softened
120g (¾ cup) chopped cashew nuts
120g (⅔ cup) raisins

Rinse the rice until the water runs clear. Put the rice in a medium saucepan with the water, cinnamon stick, cloves, bay leaves, saffron and salt. Bring to the boil, reduce the heat to low and cook, covered for 15 minutes. Remove from the heat and let sit, without removing the lid, for 10 minutes. Remove the big chunky herbs (bay, cloves, cinnamon), before gently stirring in the butter, cashews and raisins with a fork.

Cinnamon is a cleansing spice and is antimicrobial, saffron can help relieve inflammation and is an anti-depressant. Bay leaf contains eugenol, which has anti-inflammatory and antioxidant properties. Topically, bay oil can be used for bruising and sprains.

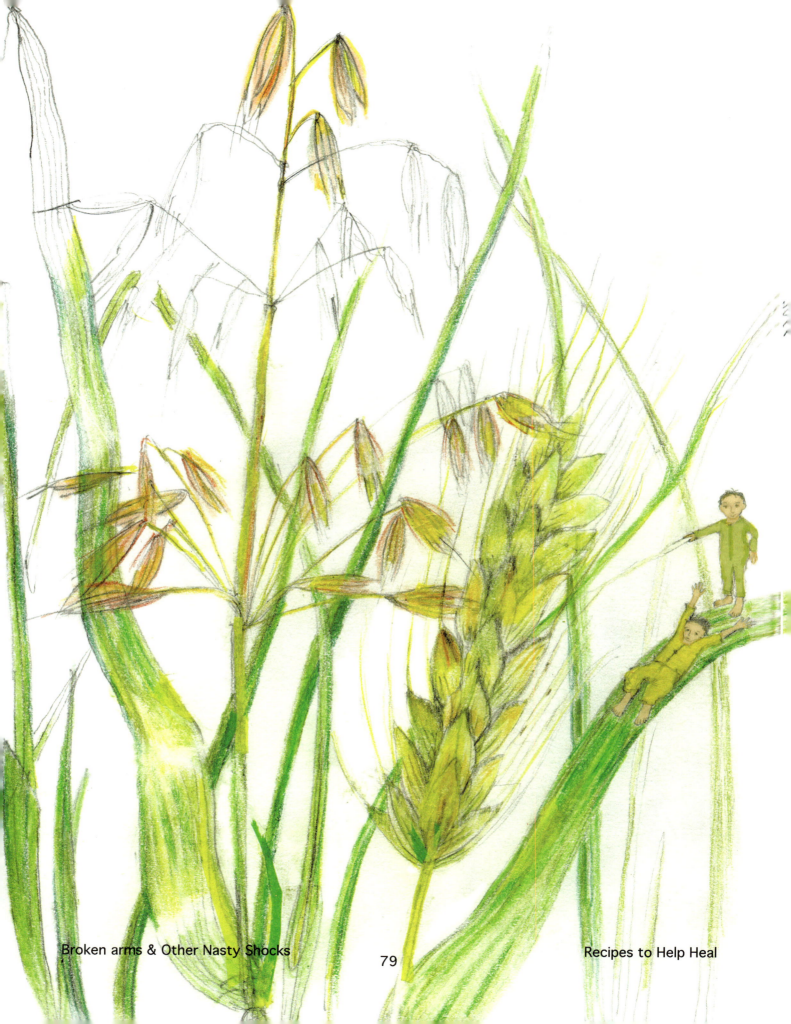

Bravery "There-There's"

100g (1 cup) each millet, rye, quinoa, oat & barley flakes
50g (⅓ cup) each sesame, pumpkin, sunflower & linseeds
50g (⅓ cup) each chopped dried peaches, pears & figs
1 tablespoon agave syrup
1 tablespoon honey
4 tablespoons sunflower oil

Warm the sunflower oil in a roasting tin. Stir in all the ingredients and bake at 180C (350F/ Gas 4) for 20 minutes, stirring occasionally. Remove from the oven and whilst still warm, roll into little balls of sweets, perfect for popping in the mouth.

The seeds provide anti-inflammatory fats, quinoa is a great source of protein, and oats and barley are calming.

Almond & Pine Nut Soup

220g (2 cups) blanched almonds
220g (2 cups) pine nuts
2 tablespoons agave syrup or honey
750ml (3 cups) coconut or almond milk
2 teaspoons ground cinnamon

Soak nuts in warm water for an hour, drain and whizz in a blender with agave or honey. Put into a saucepan, add milk, bring to the boil and sprinkle with cinnamon. Serve slightly warm.

Nuts contain lots of anti-inflammatory omega fats, which will calm down anything that is swollen, and also lots of powerful nutrients which are good for healing. Almonds are full of protein which is needed to repair and lots of vitamin E and magnesium which all help heal.

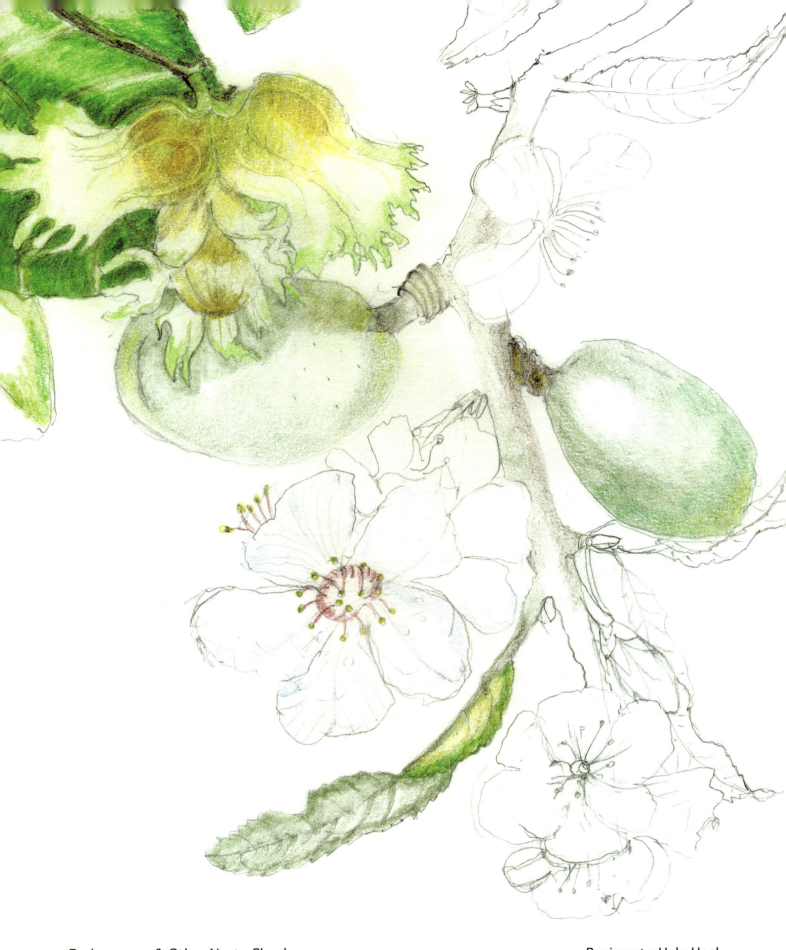

Hazelnut Shortbread

50g (2oz) skinless hazelnuts
340g (2¾ cups) chestnut flour
220g (2¼ cups) ground almonds
2 eggs
2 tablespoons agave syrup or manuka honey
2 tablespoons olive oil

Simmer the hazelnuts for half an hour in a pan of boiling water, take off the heat and leave to cool in the water. Drain and then whizz in blender until pureed.

Put the pureed hazelnuts into a bowl and add all the other ingredients, mix to a soft dough. Line a baking tray with greaseproof paper, spread the dough until about 2 centimetres thick. Bake at 220C (425F/Gas 7) for 20 minutes, until just turning golden brown - do not over cook. Remove from oven, cut into squares and serve when cool.

Chocolate & Hazelnut Gratin

220g (1 ¾ cups) rice flour
500ml (2 cups) rice milk
50g (2oz) dark chocolate
220g (2¼ cups) finely ground hazelnuts

In a medium saucepan, toast the chestnut flour over a low heat until it just starts to brown, then add the milk and chocolate (broken into small pieces), and warm over a low heat until the chocolate is melted. Remove from the heat and stir in the hazelnuts. Pour into an oiled baking dish and bake for 15 minutes at 200C (400F/Gas 6).

Hazelnuts are a rich source of omega 9 and vitamin E (which helps to heal wounds and scars), minerals and antioxidants, as well as lots of dietary fibre. Dark chocolate contains lots of antioxidants, in the form or polyphenols and catechins, (four times as many as tea), and these are thought to be highly protective - among many other things as a cough preventer and antidiarrheal.

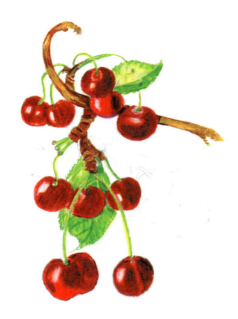

BIOFLAVONOIDS are antioxidant, antiviral & anti-inflammatory compounds which are found in many fruits & vegetables such as cherries, grapes, tea & soya.

CANTHAXANTHIN is a carotenoid which is found in mushrooms, egg yolk, green algae, crustaceans & fish. It is a potent radical scavenger & nature's most powerful fat-soluble antioxidant; it also protects vitamin E.

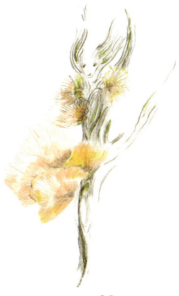

Sofa Stage & Recovery Blues

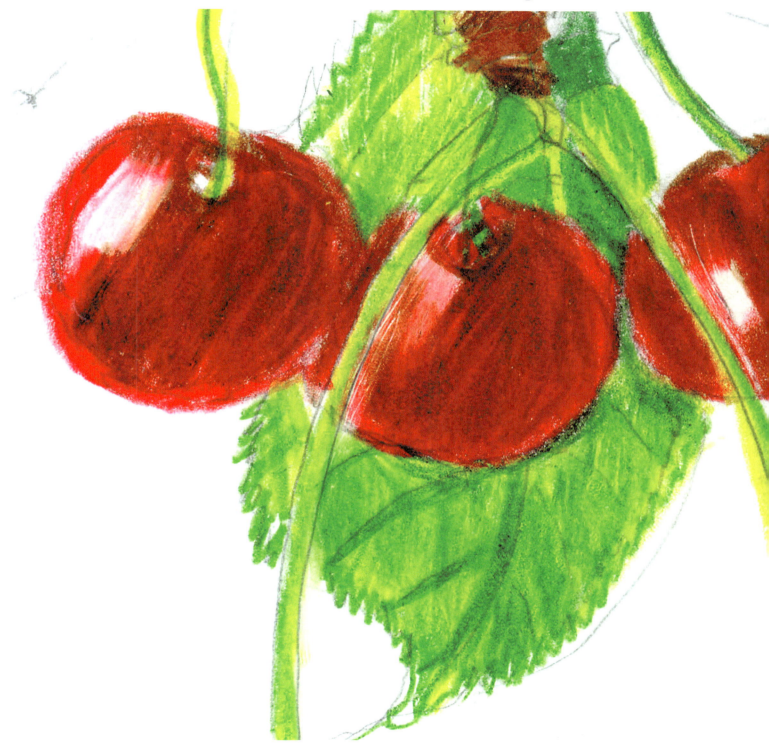

Recipes For Children to Make

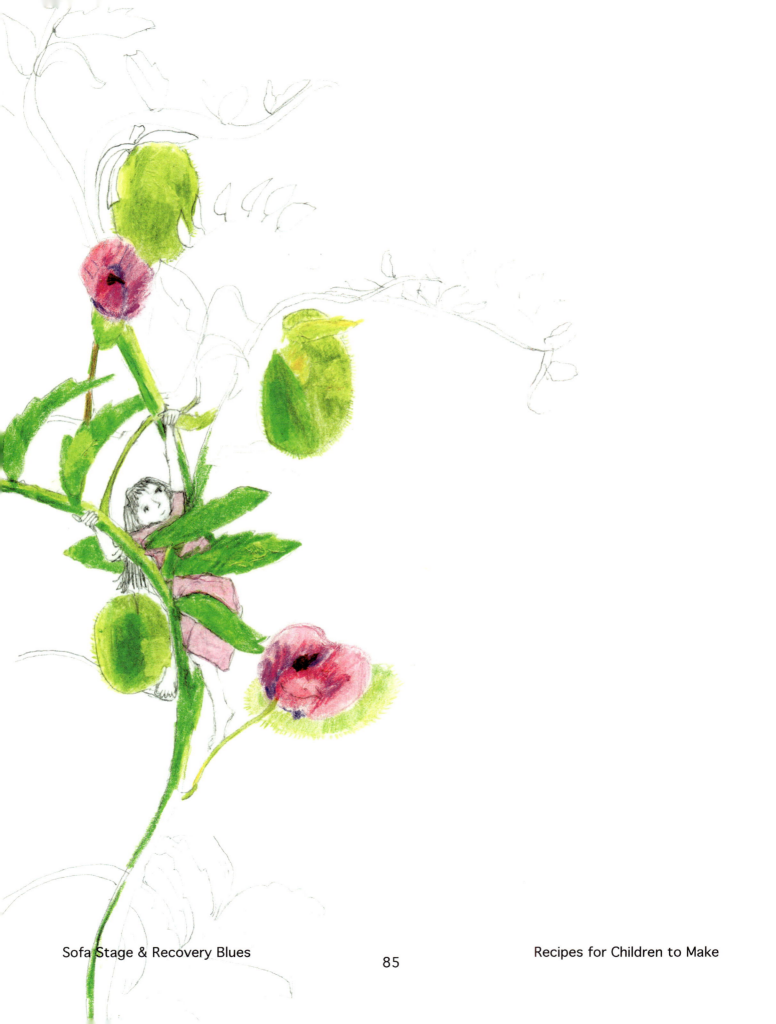

The Sofa Stage

Eventually your child will start feeling better and progress from languishing in bed being floppy and compliant, to the sofa stage. This is perhaps the most challenging as the recuperating patient is likely to be up and down with fluctuating energy levels, possibly grumpy, not quite ready for school, bored and demanding. Food needs to be calming, enticing, hydrating and mood levelling.

In this chapter, there are recipes for children to make, sweet treats without sugar highs and snack foods that are fun to eat to encourage appetite.

Falafels

400g tin chickpeas in water
1 small onion, finely chopped
6 spring onions, finely chopped
1 clove of garlic, crushed
½ teaspoon ground cumin
1 teaspoon ground coriander seeds
½ teaspoon baking powder
1 egg (optional)
3 tablespoons olive oil

Preheat oven to 220C (425F/Gas7). Heat half the oil in a shallow baking tray. Grind to a paste, (in a blender or food processor), all the ingredients apart from the egg and the oil. Add the egg if the mixture looks too dry to make into balls. Roll the falafel mixture in your hands into walnut-sized balls, and then flatten slightly. Heat the remaining oil in a frying pan and fry the falafel balls on a high heat, turning often until sides are sealed. Remove from frying pan and place in shallow baking tray and then roast for 10 to 15 minutes, shaking the dish often until browned on all sides. Drain on kitchen paper before serving.

Chickpeas have a gel-like soluble fibre which slows down the release of blood sugar, meaning that energy is sustained at a steady level rather than peaking and troughing.

Chickpea Dip

400g tin chickpeas, drained & rinsed
2 tablespoons sesame seed paste/ tahini
3 tablespoons live Greek-style yogurt
1 clove garlic
juice of 1 lemon
handful basil and mint leaves
4 tablespoons olive, hempseed or linseed oil
   (whichever you prefer the taste of)

Whizz everything except the oil into a blender. Gradually pour in the oil until the preferred consistency/smoothness is reached. If too gloopy, add a little cold water and whizz again.

Beetroot Hummus

2 raw beetroot, washed, peeled & grated
1 tin chickpeas, drained & rinsed
1 pinch salt
juice of 1 lemon
1 garlic clove, crushed
4 tablespoons natural yogurt
1 tablespoon extra virgin olive oil
4 wholemeal pitta breads
1 cucumber, 1 carrot, 1 pepper, to serve

Place all the ingredients except the pitta and vegetable sticks into a food processor or blender and whizz until pureed. Transfer to a bowl and serve with warm pitta bread and sticks of cucumber, carrot and pepper.

Beetroot is packed with vitamins and it makes the hummus turn bright pink, giving it a real "wow" factor. Encourage children to help by peeling and grating the beetroot, washing the vegetables and operating the food processor or blender with adult supervision.

Avocado Dip - See Chapter 5

Any leftover dips - make like Jim Carey and "The Mask". Choose a favourite DVD and slather your face with smashed avocado or beetroot dip. Perfect for your skin and fun to do with a bored child who wants company. Obviously protect your furniture/clothes with tea towels and paste on carefully. Leave for about 20 minutes.

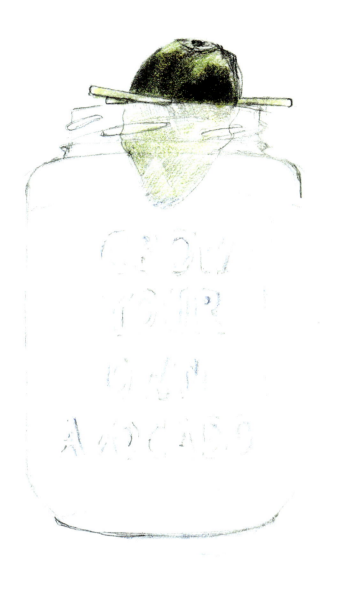

Eat an avocado and save the stone. Fill a jam jar with water. Take four toothpicks and pierce into the stone at the four "corners" so that the avocado can balance over the jar rim and the water just covers the pointy bottom. Keep topped up with water and eventually you will have an avocado plant. It may not produce avocados, but it is a handsome plant with glossy leaves.

Take a garlic bulb and pick off individual cloves. Plant them outside in Autumn or early Spring. Plant with the pointy end upwards in a hole deep enough to leave the top just covered. Each clove will grow into a bulb of garlic by Summer.

Sushi

Sushi Rice

160g (1 cup) sushi rice
400ml (1½ cups) of water
splodge of Japanese rice wine
dollop of Japanese vinegar
sprinkle of sugar & salt

Bring the rice to the boil and allow to cook for 10 minutes at quite a high heat, in a pan with a firm lid. Put the other ingredients into a small bowl, mix together and evenly pour over the rice. Leave for 10 minutes and gently stir.

Sushi Maki

1 sheet nori seaweed
packet of smoked salmon
sushi rice as above
bamboo rolling mat

Place the nori seaweed on the bamboo rolling mat. Dip hands in cold water, (this stops the rice sticking to you), and put a 1cm thick square of rice on the nori with a 1cm border around it. Slightly north of the middle, place strips of smoked salmon. Using the rolling mat, roll towards you keeping the roll tight. When you have rolled into a sausage shape, carefully cut into rounds.

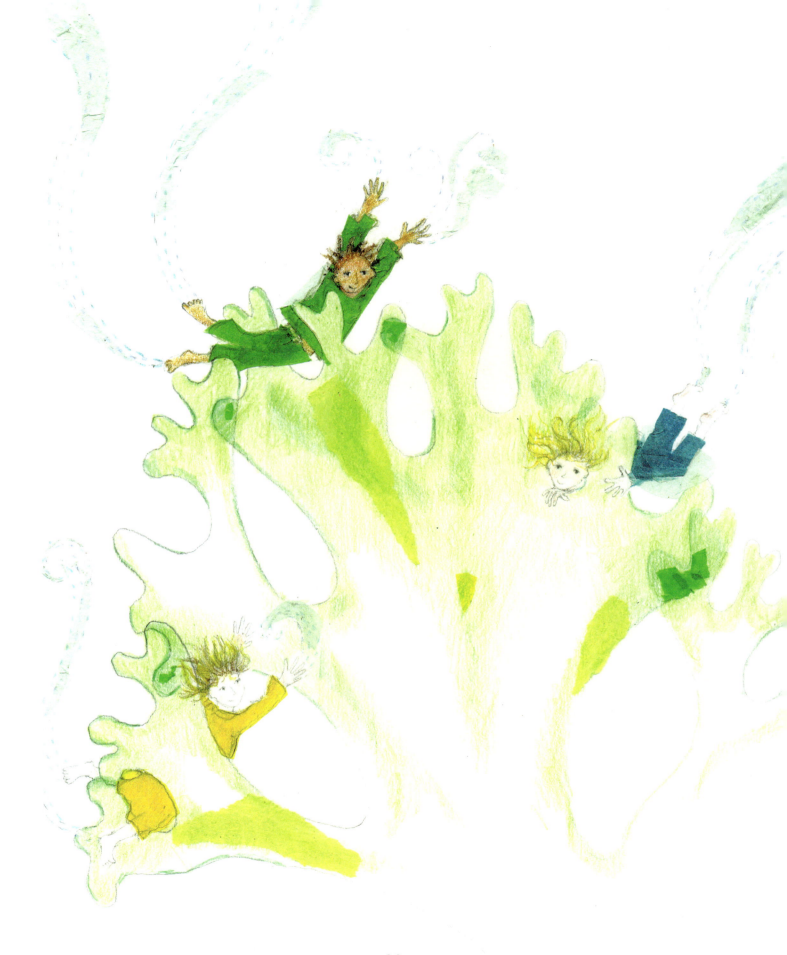

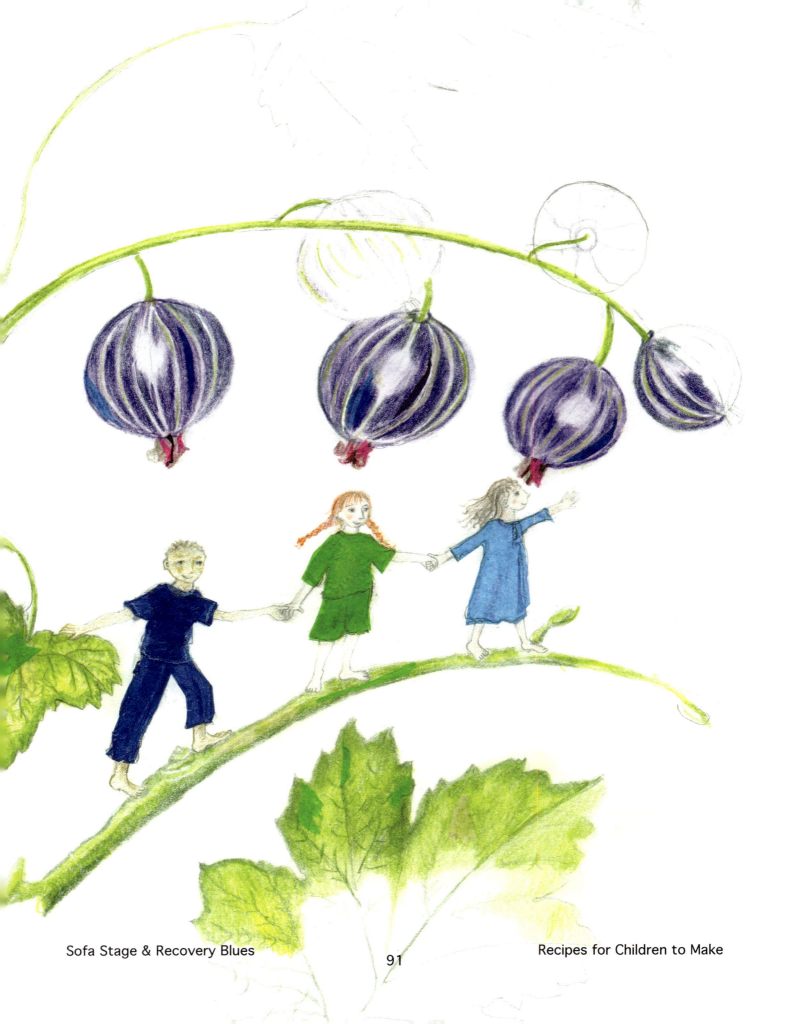

Blackcurrant Syrup

250g (8½ oz) blackcurrants, washed
60g (¾ cup) xylitol or fructose sugar
200ml (¾ cup) water

Place the blackcurrants and 200ml of water in a saucepan and bring to the boil. Simmer for 10 minutes, squashing the blackcurrants with a wooden spoon occasionally.
Remove from the heat and press through a sieve, add the sugar whilst the syrup is still warm and stir until all the sugar has dissolved. Pour into a sterilised screw top jar, cool and keep in the fridge for up to two weeks.

This syrup is good mixed with sparkling water or natural yogurt. You can ask children to top and tail the blackcurrants if you need to keep them occupied.

Home-made Tomato Ketchup

1 kg (2lb) organic vine tomatoes
3 teaspoons tarragon wine vinegar
3 tablespoons xylitol or fructose sugar
2 pinches cinnamon, ground mace & allspice
2 pinches ground black pepper
2 pinches sea salt

Roughly chop the tomatoes, place in a pan with 2 tablespoons of water. Cook for 5 minutes, stirring, and when cool, liquidize and sieve. Return to the pan and stir in the vinegar, sugar and spices. Bring to the boil and simmer until it reaches a thick tomato sauce consistency, then pour into a sterilised bottle.

Orange & Almond Cake

This lovely cake is dairy and wheat free so is easy on the body, and with the sugar replacement, it won't give your blood sugar a turbo-boost, so should help keep you steady.

1 medium orange
150g (¾ cup/5oz) xylitol or steva sugar replacement
3 eggs
250g (2½ cups/8oz) ground almonds
½ teaspoon baking powder

Use two 8 inch round tins, oiled and lined with baking paper. Preheat oven to 180C (350F/Gas 4).

Put the orange in a saucepan, cover with water, bring to the boil and then simmer for a minute. Remove from the pan and when it is cool enough to handle, cut orange in half. Take pips out and whizz in the food processor or blender. Whisk eggs and sugar until thick and pale, then fold in the almonds, orange and baking powder. Pour into tins and cook for 45 to 50 minutes. Let the cake cool in the tin. Serve with bioactive Greek yogurt. Delicious with sliced oranges as a pudding.

Use peeled pineapple instead of orange to suppress inflammation, or berries (blueberry, blackberry, cranberry, strawberry) for a super antioxidant cake.

Almonds are rich in vitamin E and antioxidants, and also calcium, which promotes growth and muscle strength.

Oranges are a reliable source of vitamin C which sustains the body's resistance to infection and its ability to heal. Flavonoids found in the skin of an orange support vitamin C action. They are also a good source of potassium which helps regulate fluid levels in the body, which can be disrupted by some medications.

Bioactive yogurt does not have the same inflammatory properties as other dairy products, and it provides essential probiotics which help the gut, protect against upset stomachs and support the immune system, especially if antibiotics have been taken.

Eggs are a good source of protein (to build you up), selenium (to protect you), iodine, B vitamins, iron, zinc and vitamins D and E.

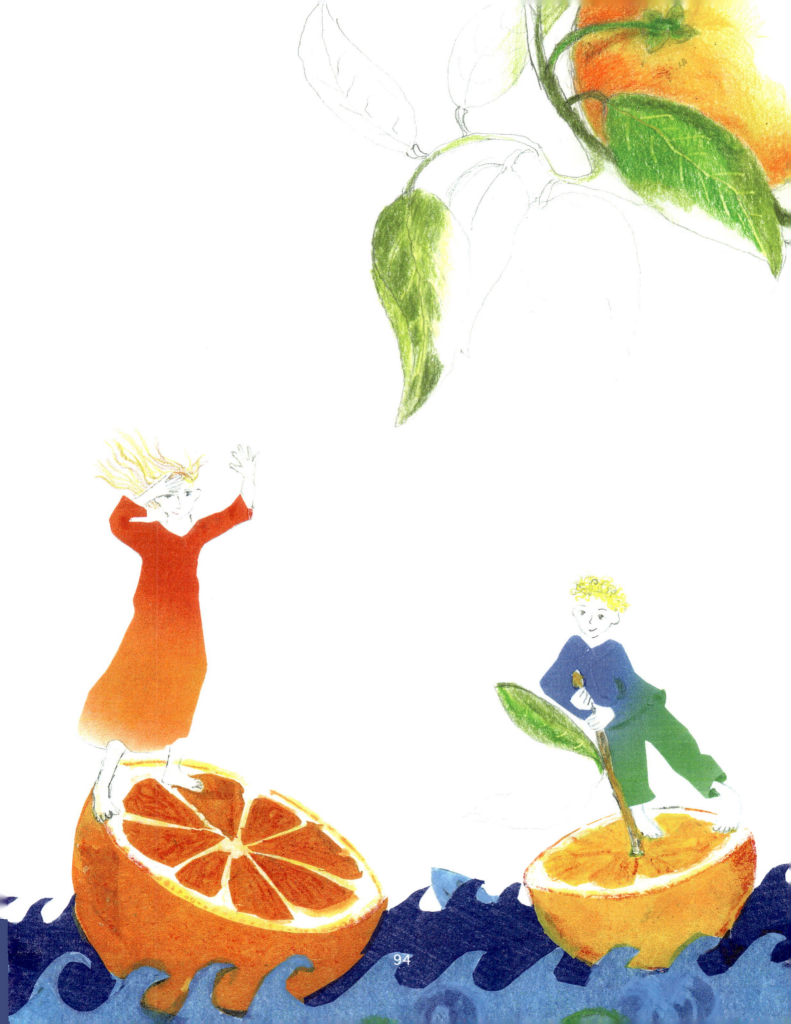

Fruity Papyrus

500g (1lb) apricots, peaches, nectarines or berries
500g (1lb) eating apples, peeled & chopped
juice of 1 lemon
150g (½ cup) runny manuka honey

In a saucepan bring all the ingredients to the boil and then a low simmer. Cover and cook gently for 20 minutes until pulpy. Allow to cool a little, then push through a sieve with the back of a spoon. Line two baking sheets with baking parchment. Divide the puree between the two baking trays, tip to spread the mixture to the edge.

Put in the oven at a low temperature, 70C (150F/Gas 1). Bake for 8 to 10 hours, until slightly tacky and easy to peel from the paper. When cool, cut into strips.

This is a great after-school snack, or sweet pick-me-up, and it is easy and fun to make.

Other quick and easy recovery meals to cook with children include fish cakes, chicken wrapped in wheat free tortillas, smoked salmon and scrambled eggs, quiche, spring rolls, pizzas.

Dipping fruit in chocolate is also fun and healthy.

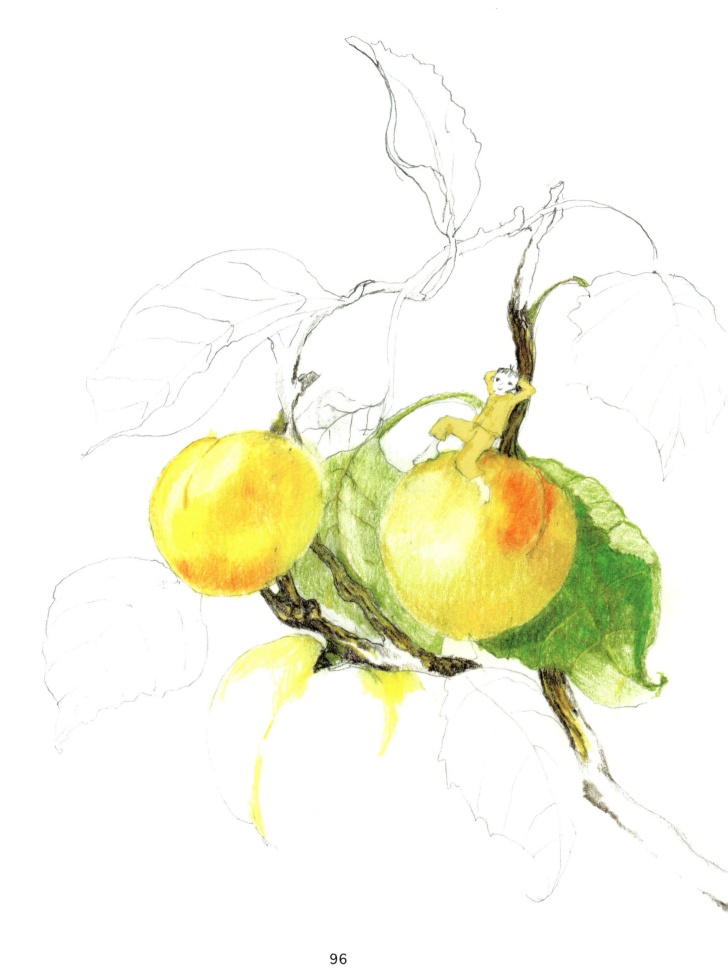

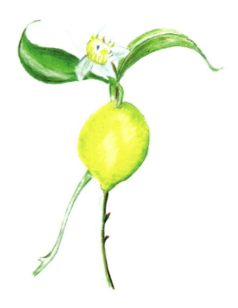

HESPERIDIN is the flavonoid found in lots
of citrus fruits like oranges, tangerines,
grapefruits, clementines, lemons, limes,
mandarins, pomelos, kumquats, ugli fruits
& tangelos. It is an antioxidant,
anti-inflammatory & a natural sedative.

Quick Cures for Little Sores

A First Aid Kit for Small Emergencies
or Persistant Problems

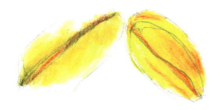

Allergic Reactions

Parsley contains vitamins A and C which help reduce reactions.

Drink elderflower tea.

Anxiety, Exam Stress

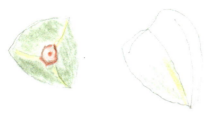

Drink lemon balm, valerian or jasmine flower tea or add to bath, anti-depressant & relaxing.

Add oats & rosemary to diet.

Bruising

Put 20 drops of essential oil of lavender in 2 teaspoons of carrier oil. This can be rubbed onto bruises & cuts to help them heal.

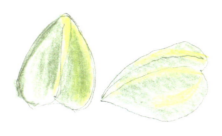

Lettuce or cabbage leaves can be applied directly to bruises to help remove inflammation, just bind to area & change every few hours.

Arnica ointment is good for bruising, make sure there are no cuts as arnica should not enter the blood stream.

Chop a handful of parsley, add to hot water, boil for 5 minutes, leave until lukewarm, strain, apply with cotton wool to bruise.

Eat blueberries or bilberries.

Burns (minor)

Cut leaf from aloe vera plant 7.5cm from tip. On a work surface using a sharp knife, slice up to middle of leaf, peel back the sides to expose clear gel inside, (not the yellow sap released on the side of the leaf). Apply to skin for minor burns - after 10 minutes under cold running water. Do not apply to open wounds.

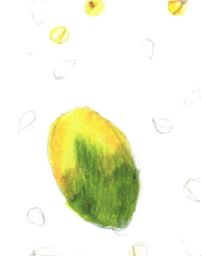

Add 5 drops of lavender essential oil to a base oil, and apply with cotton wool.

Use pumpkin fruit pulp as a poultice.

Mashed avocado will help to heal the burn.

Cold Sores

Cold sores are caused by a virus, so any antiviral remedy will have some effect. The lysine in beans, chicken and lamb can prevent the virus from spreading. Avoid arginine, found in chocolate, coconut, peanuts, oats & wheat.

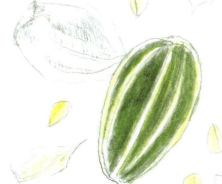

Apply vitamin E capsules directly onto the cold sore to help heal. Tea tree oil can be used topically as it is strongly antiviral, as can manuka honey.

Aloe vera gel can be cooling.

Quick cures for little sores

Colds, Catarrh, Chest Infections

Drink elderflower as a cordial or tisane.

Drink rosemary tisane.

Make a cinnamon tea (steep 2 sticks in hot water). Drink 3 times a day for convalescence.

Blackberry juice is particularly good for colds.

Steam inhaler - make a "tea" with thyme, camomile & rosemary. Add to a bowl of hot water with tea tree or eucalyptus oil. Put a towel over head & breath in deeply.

Infuse an onion slice in hot water for a few minutes to make a drink which relieves runny noses.

Convalescence

Drink nettle tea; cover fresh young shoots with hot water & infuse for 10 minutes.

For soup: steam nettles, add to cooked carrots & onions, cover with hot water, simmer for 5 minutes, add a knob of butter & blend.

Add beetroot & carrot juice to coconut milk. This drink will act as a cleanser.

Dandelion salad with marigold & borage flowers is a good tonic.

Barley is very good for convalescence either eaten as a food or drunk as barley water.

Coughs

Infuse caraway seeds to make a soothing tea.

Nasturtium infusion is good for chest infections as it contains lots of vitamin C.

Nasturtium leaves & flowers can also be used in salads.

Earache

Drinking warm elderflower juice, blackcurrant juice or lemon & honey will soothe the pain.

Press a warm hot water bottle against ear.

Add garlic, turmeric & ginger to diet.

There are appropriate probiotics for glue ear.

Fevers

Strong mint tea will induce perspiration.

Watermelon soothes a feverish throat.

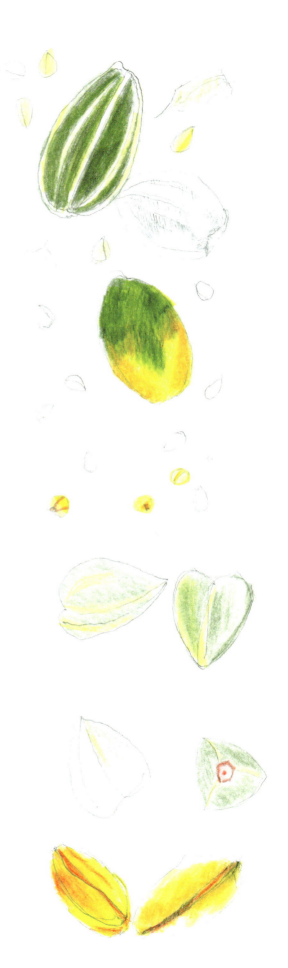

Head Lice

Add essential oil of tea tree, lavender, eucalyptus & rosemary to a few drops of carrier oil. Rub onto scalp or put in water & spray on hair.

Staphisagria is a homeopathic remedy which can be used to prevent re-infestation.

Motion Sickness

Drink ginger, camomile or lemon balm tea.

Mouth Ulcers

Dab aloe vera gel in mouth on ulcers or aching teeth.

Rub with a basil leaf.

Gargle with a herbal tea.

Nappy Rash

Bathe bottom in herbal infusion of lavender, marigold & camomile.

St John's wort oil, calendula oil & rose water also help.

Calendula cream can help heal & protect skin.

Nose Bleeds

Sit down & lean head forward (not back). Eat lots of vitamin C and bioflavonoids (found in all fruit & vegetables) to help build capillary walls.

To stop bleeding, apply a cold compress (e.g. small bag of frozen peas) or soak cotton wool with witch hazel & hold against nose.

Arnica & Phosphorus are useful homeopathic remedies for nose bleeds.

Sore Eyes

Drink raspberry leaf tea infusion.

Add a few drops of euphrasia tincture to water & drink.

Place slices of cucumber on the eyes.

Styes are a bacteria infection at the root of an eyelash - use euphrasia as a tincture or infusion. Put onto cotton wool as a compress. Pulsatilla is a useful homeopathic remedy if stye is filled with pus.

Conjunctivitis is inflammation of the membrane covering the eyeball. Bathe the eye at least 3 times a day with 5 drops of rosewater & 5 drops of euphrasia in ½ cup of warm water. You can also make a herbal compress with camomile or fennel tea bags.

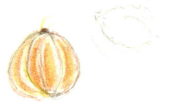

Quick cures for little sores

Sore Throats

Make rosemary leaves into a tisane or tea.

Suck frozen blackberries (halved).

Make herb and honey ice cubes to suck.

Gargle with sage tea or blackberry leaf tea as a mouthwash.

Eat barley - as a porridge/ pudding or barley water.

Stings & Bites

Rub aloe vera gel & sage leaves on bite or sting.

Toothache

Chew tarragon or oregano leaves.

Chew cloves.

Star anise - either suck or use as a tea or gargle.

For teething: cold yoghurt can soothe, gently massage on gum. Also biting on a carrot or apple kept in the fridge - hard & cold.

Urinary Tract Infections

Take rosehip syrup.

Drink vervain tea (also stimulates poor appetite).

Unsweetened cranberry juice - use apple or orange juice to sweeten. Drink 1 litre (4 cups) a day for a few days.

Drink lemon barley water.

Eat kava kava (can settle irritable bowel too).

Worms

Drink thyme tea or add thyme to food.

Add garlic to food.

Eat raw carrot root grated - a safe treatment for threadworms.

Ground pumpkin seeds with water, milk and honey are helpful against worms & tapeworms.

Eat pumpkin nut butter.

Whizz up watermelon flesh with the seeds in a blender. Add ice cubes to make a cool drink.

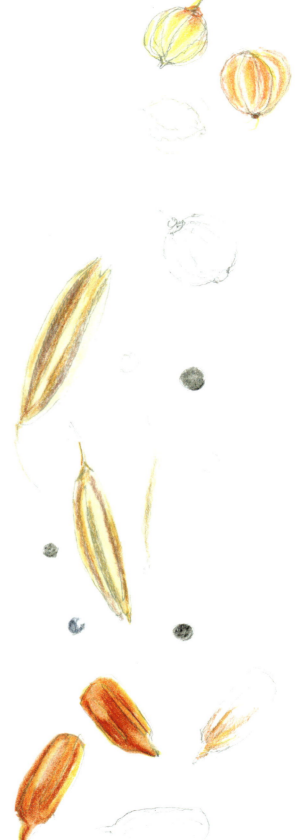

Index

Index

What is the immune system?

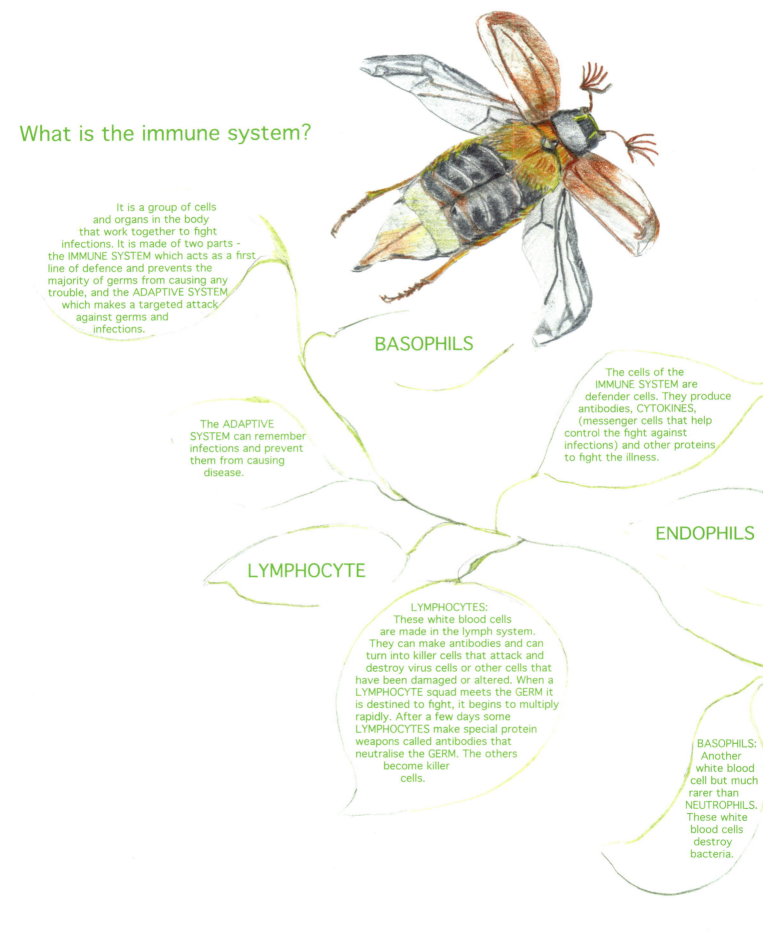

It is a group of cells and organs in the body that work together to fight infections. It is made of two parts - the IMMUNE SYSTEM which acts as a first line of defence and prevents the majority of germs from causing any trouble, and the ADAPTIVE SYSTEM which makes a targeted attack against germs and infections.

BASOPHILS

The cells of the IMMUNE SYSTEM are defender cells. They produce antibodies, CYTOKINES, (messenger cells that help control the fight against infections) and other proteins to fight the illness.

The ADAPTIVE SYSTEM can remember infections and prevent them from causing disease.

ENDOPHILS

LYMPHOCYTE

LYMPHOCYTES:
These white blood cells are made in the lymph system. They can make antibodies and can turn into killer cells that attack and destroy virus cells or other cells that have been damaged or altered. When a LYMPHOCYTE squad meets the GERM it is destined to fight, it begins to multiply rapidly. After a few days some LYMPHOCYTES make special protein weapons called antibodies that neutralise the GERM. The others become killer cells.

BASOPHILS:
Another white blood cell but much rarer than NEUTROPHILS. These white blood cells destroy bacteria.

105

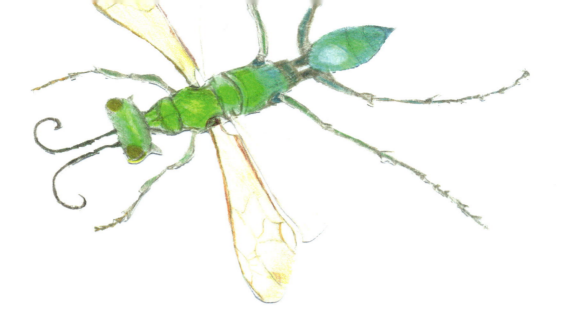

ENDOPHILS:
This white blood cell circulates in the blood and kills the larvae of parasitic worms that invade cells in your body, but if your body is under an allergic attack, they are powerful weapons.

NEUTROPHILS

MACROPHAGES:
They engulf and destroy enemy cells, help LYMPHOCYTES make antibodies and killer cells and clear up debris NEUTROPHILS. Made up in the bone marrow, these white blood cells gobble up and destroy invading GERMS. You make up to 80 million in a minute.

MACROPHAGES

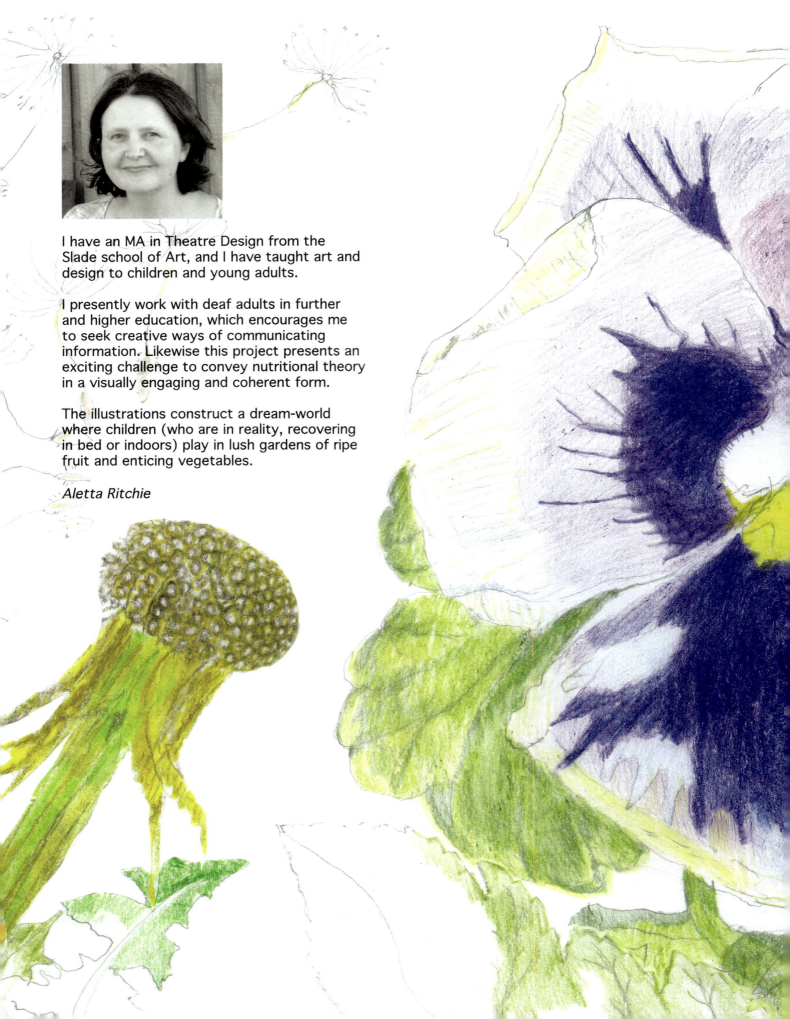

I have an MA in Theatre Design from the Slade school of Art, and I have taught art and design to children and young adults.

I presently work with deaf adults in further and higher education, which encourages me to seek creative ways of communicating information. Likewise this project presents an exciting challenge to convey nutritional theory in a visually engaging and coherent form.

The illustrations construct a dream-world where children (who are in reality, recovering in bed or indoors) play in lush gardens of ripe fruit and enticing vegetables.

Aletta Ritchie

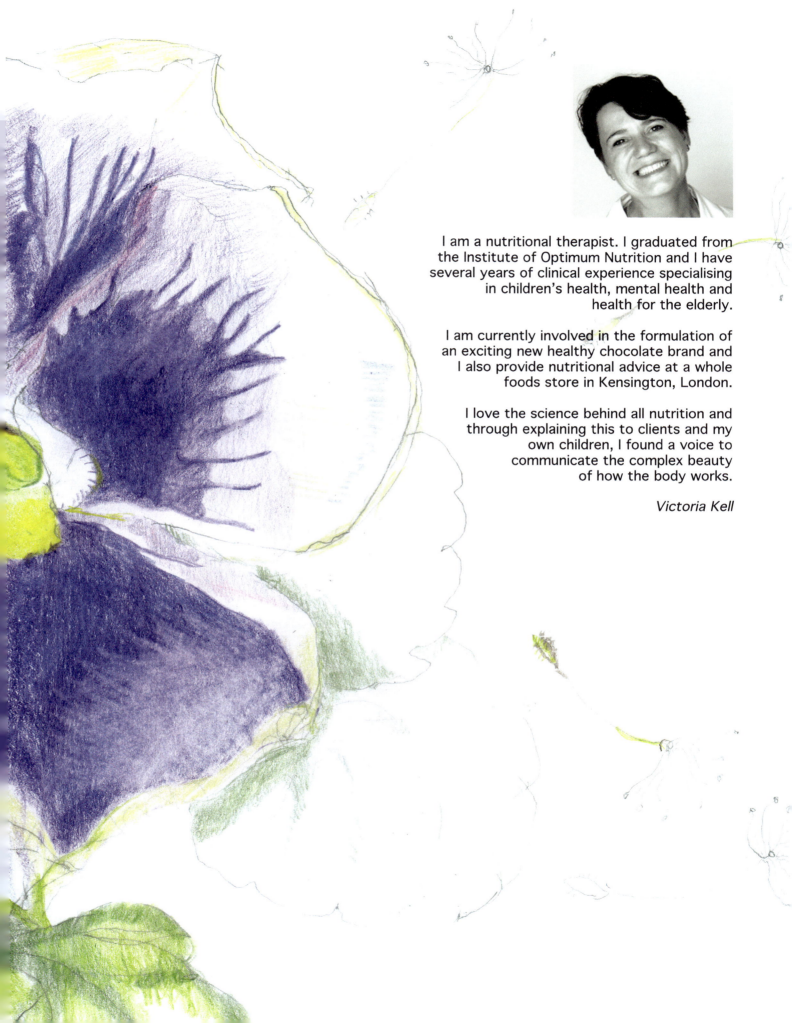

I am a nutritional therapist. I graduated from the Institute of Optimum Nutrition and I have several years of clinical experience specialising in children's health, mental health and health for the elderly.

I am currently involved in the formulation of an exciting new healthy chocolate brand and I also provide nutritional advice at a whole foods store in Kensington, London.

I love the science behind all nutrition and through explaining this to clients and my own children, I found a voice to communicate the complex beauty of how the body works.

Victoria Kell

Lightning Source UK Ltd.
Milton Keynes UK
UKIC01n2248010515
250764UK00006B/25